CARDIOLOGY RESEARCH AND CLINICAL DEVELOPMENTS

AORTIC ANEURYSMS

SIGNS, SYMPTOMS AND MANAGEMENT

CARDIOLOGY RESEARCH AND CLINICAL DEVELOPMENTS

Additional books and e-books in this series can be found on Nova's website under the Series tab.

CARDIOLOGY RESEARCH AND CLINICAL DEVELOPMENTS

AORTIC ANEURYSMS

SIGNS, SYMPTOMS AND MANAGEMENT

AMER HARKY
EDITOR

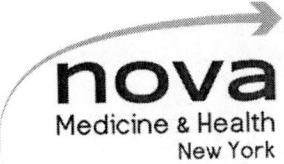

Copyright © 2020 by Nova Science Publishers, Inc.

All rights reserved. No part of this book may be reproduced, stored in a retrieval system or transmitted in any form or by any means: electronic, electrostatic, magnetic, tape, mechanical photocopying, recording or otherwise without the written permission of the Publisher.

We have partnered with Copyright Clearance Center to make it easy for you to obtain permissions to reuse content from this publication. Simply navigate to this publication's page on Nova's website and locate the "Get Permission" button below the title description. This button is linked directly to the title's permission page on copyright.com. Alternatively, you can visit copyright.com and search by title, ISBN, or ISSN.

For further questions about using the service on copyright.com, please contact:
Copyright Clearance Center
Phone: +1-(978) 750-8400   Fax: +1-(978) 750-4470   E-mail: info@copyright.com.

NOTICE TO THE READER

The Publisher has taken reasonable care in the preparation of this book, but makes no expressed or implied warranty of any kind and assumes no responsibility for any errors or omissions. No liability is assumed for incidental or consequential damages in connection with or arising out of information contained in this book. The Publisher shall not be liable for any special, consequential, or exemplary damages resulting, in whole or in part, from the readers' use of, or reliance upon, this material. Any parts of this book based on government reports are so indicated and copyright is claimed for those parts to the extent applicable to compilations of such works.

Independent verification should be sought for any data, advice or recommendations contained in this book. In addition, no responsibility is assumed by the Publisher for any injury and/or damage to persons or property arising from any methods, products, instructions, ideas or otherwise contained in this publication.

This publication is designed to provide accurate and authoritative information with regard to the subject matter covered herein. It is sold with the clear understanding that the Publisher is not engaged in rendering legal or any other professional services. If legal or any other expert assistance is required, the services of a competent person should be sought. FROM A DECLARATION OF PARTICIPANTS JOINTLY ADOPTED BY A COMMITTEE OF THE AMERICAN BAR ASSOCIATION AND A COMMITTEE OF PUBLISHERS.

Additional color graphics may be available in the e-book version of this book.

Library of Congress Cataloging-in-Publication Data

ISBN: 978-1-53617-677-3
Identifiers: LCCN 2020011887 (print) | LCCN 2020011888 (ebook) | ISBN 9781536176773 (paperback) | ISBN 9781536176919 (adobe pdf)
Subjects: LCSH: Aortic aneurysms.
Classification: LCC RC693 .A564 2020 (print) | LCC RC693 (ebook) | DDC 616.1/33--dc23
LC record available at https://lccn.loc.gov/2020011887
LC ebook record available at https://lccn.loc.gov/2020011888

Published by Nova Science Publishers, Inc. † New York

CONTENTS

Preface		vii
Chapter 1	Immunopathology of Aortic Aneurysms *Ka Siu Fan, Ka Hay Fan, Hiu Tat Kwok and Amer Harky*	1
Chapter 2	Endovascular Stent Grafting of Thoracic Aortic Aneurysm *Chi Wei Ong, Foad Kabinejadian, Ala Elhelali and Hwa Liang Leo*	63
Chapter 3	Abdominal Aortic Aneurysms: Morphology, Risk Factors, Management and Image-Based Modeling Strategies *Golnaz Jalalahmadi, María Helguera and Cristian A. Linte*	109
Editor's Contact Information		149
Index		151

PREFACE

This book highlights the current importance of aortic aneurysms, their clinical presentations and methods of management. The book focuses on different segments of the aorta from the aortic root to the abdominal aorta. Not only are the clinical and pathological conditions included in this book, but also the basic immunopathology of the aortic aneurysms are thoroughly discussed.

The authors highlight the importance of the understanding the basic pathophysiology of the aneurysm formation, presentation and therefore management of each pathology. The presentation of each aortic segment aneurysm varies depending on the acute pathology. There are often such cases when these aneurysms are found accidentally while the patients are being scanned for other non-aortic conditions.

Throughout the chapters of this book, the authors have aimed to simplify the understanding of the aortic aneurysm, its clinical manifestations and methods of diagnosis and options of surgical interventions in each case.

This book serves as an important tool for those who have a special interest in aortic surgery.

Chapter 1 - From the aortic root through to abdominal aorta, aneurysm can occur at any point along the length of the aorta. They are increasingly common degenerative vascular diseases with high mortality and morbidity, primarily affecting ageing population. Despite advances in aneurysm repair, many remains asymptomatic until presented as emergency cases in the form of rupture or dissection. Pathophysiology of aneurysms are characterised by an inflammatory state mediated by secretion of proinflammatory molecules and inflammatory immune cells. These processes increase both metalloproteinases and vascular smooth muscle cell apoptosis which compromises aortic wall integrity. Additionally, dysfunctional leukocyte and lymphocyte response lead to inappropriate immunoglobulin binding and complement activation also affect disease progression. The complex interaction between cellular and molecular components lead to transmural degeneration, decrease in vascular smooth muscle cells and a chronic inflammatory state, eventually developing into an aneurysm.

The authors discussed the role of inflammatory cells, molecules and mechanisms of aortic aneurysms to better understand their underlying immunopathology. With improved understanding, there may be both therapeutic and preventative potential in immunotherapy as an alternative to surgical repairs.

Chapter 2 - Thoracic aortic aneurysm (TAA) can be a silent killer if left untreated. Open surgery needs a longer recovery process and is not suitable for high-risk patients. Thoracic endovascular aortic repair (TEVAR) has been introduced as a less invasive approach to management of thoracic aortic aneurysm (TAA). Common TEVAR approaches involve implantation of a simple Dacron stent graft through a catheter. However, the effectiveness of TEVAR in the management of TAA is often limited by the complex anatomy of the aortic arch. Branched and fenestrated stent grafts have been developed to preserve perfusion of superior branches with a low incidence of sealing zone failure. The disadvantage of the branched and fenestrated techniques is that they require custom-made devices and complex procedures, which make them less promising in urgent TEVAR. Moreover, the branched and fenestrated stent grafts have been shown to be prone to proximal endoleak that could lead to increased mortality. Another novel technique is called chimney technique. Chimney technique is a stent placed parallel to the aortic stent graft to preserve the blood flow to superior branches that was overstented to achieve an adequate seal. Even though the technique outcome is encouraging, it is difficult to fabricate a dedicated covered stent for chimney repair.

In this chapter, the authors will discuss the novel stenting technique for TAA which applies engineering fluid mechanics knowledge on the innovation of medical device. Innovative devices such as the multilayer flow modulator (MFM) have recently been proposed to provide an alternative endovascular treatment. The main purpose of MFM is to decrease the risk of rupture by modulating the flow pattern which can then lead to a reduction in local shear stress along the weakened artery wall. The authors will evaluate the pros and cons of disruptive technologies such as MFM and compare them with the above-mentioned methods such as conventional TEVAR, fenestrated, and chimney repair. An overview of the elective and emergency approach using MFM and other innovative approaches published in the existing literature will be discussed. This review indicates that although most of the innovative techniques appear to be successful, the expansion of aneurysm does not slow down immediately, and usually, only a short period of follow up results are presented. These innovations will require more clinical trials and longer follow up studies to confirm the feasibility of this disruptive technology. The presented review in this chapter can provide great insight into the nature, diagnosis, and potential improvements for the intervention involving TAA.

Chapter 3 - Abdominal aortic aneurysms (AAAs) are degenerative expansions of the infra-renal region of aorta. It has been suggested that various types of parameters contribute to the weakening of the vessel wall and growth of the AAA, eventually leading to fatal AAA rupture. In this chapter, the authors review the AAA morphology and the three main categories of parameters that influence AAA behavior, including geometrical indices, biomechanical parameters, and lifestyle and health history. The authors also review different strategies for monitoring and managing AAA progression, and available treatment options.

In: Aortic Aneurysms
Editor: Amer Harky

ISBN: 978-1-53617-677-3
© 2020 Nova Science Publishers, Inc.

Chapter 1

IMMUNOPATHOLOGY OF AORTIC ANEURYSMS

Ka Siu Fan[1],*, Ka Hay Fan[2],
Hiu Tat Kwok[3] and Amer Harky[4]

[1]St. George's Medical School, University of London, London, UK
[2]Faculty of Medicine, Imperial College London, London, UK
[3]Leicester Medical School, Leicester, UK
[4]Department of Cardiothoracic Surgery, Liverpool Heart and Chest, Liverpool, UK

ABSTRACT

From the aortic root through to abdominal aorta, aneurysm can occur at any point along the length of the aorta. They are increasingly common degenerative vascular diseases with high mortality and morbidity, primarily affecting ageing population. Despite advances in aneurysm repair, many remains asymptomatic until presented as emergency cases in the form of rupture or dissection. Pathophysiology of aneurysms are characterised by an inflammatory state mediated by secretion of proinflammatory molecules and inflammatory immune cells. These

* Corresponding Author's Email: fankasiu@gmail.com.

processes increase both metalloproteinases and vascular smooth muscle cell apoptosis which compromises aortic wall integrity. Additionally, dysfunctional leukocyte and lymphocyte response lead to inappropriate immunoglobulin binding and complement activation also affect disease progression. The complex interaction between cellular and molecular components lead to transmural degeneration, decrease in vascular smooth muscle cells and a chronic inflammatory state, eventually developing into an aneurysm.

We discussed the role of inflammatory cells, molecules and mechanisms of aortic aneurysms to better understand their underlying immunopathology. With improved understanding, there may be both therapeutic and preventative potential in immunotherapy as an alternative to surgical repairs.

Keywords: immunopathology, aortic aneurysm, inflammation, degeneration

INTRODUCTION

Population ageing has been and will continue to remain a global challenge to healthcare as a whole; while currently 11% of the global population is over 60 years of age, it is expected to increase to 22% by 2050 [1]. As evident across many studies, ageing presents a major risk factor for various cardiovascular diseases [2,3]. While ageing introduces structural and functional changes to the heart, the aorta undergoes a myriad of changes.

Aortic aneurysms are pathological dilation of aorta greater than 1.5 times its normal size and is an increasingly prevalent disease [4]. Despite advances, contribution of ageing has raised the global aortic aneurysm deaths from 2.49 to 2.78 per 100,000 over the past decades [5]. With most cases asymptomatic, they typically remain undetected where they continue to grow in size until it rupture, where mortality rates often exceed 90% [6]. To date, surgery remains the only viable intervention and a better understanding of its pathophysiology may allow development of novel therapeutics [7,8].

Currently, even with knowledge of its atherosclerotic and genetic aetiology, AA remains a multifactorial disease with much of its underlying mechanics still yet to be discovered. Like in atherosclerotic changes, our immune system is believed to be involved throughout the development of aortic aneurysms through various facets, including pro-inflammatory changes and auto-immunity. This chapter sets out to explore these processes in the context of effector cells, their molecular actions and involvement of various receptors.

DISCUSSION

To understand the complex pathophysiology of aortic aneurysms, we must understand the aorta and its normal physiological changes that occur during ageing. The aorta is comprised of several layers, with the innermost tunica intima, intima media and tunica externa/adventitia outermost [9]. The tunica intima is a single layer of endothelial cells on a basement membrane and serves to provide optimal fluid dynamics for non-thrombogenic surface blood flow. Tunica media is the middle layer containing elastic fibres and vascular smooth muscle cells (VSMC) arranged in a lamellar structure to allow appropriate expansion or contraction in accordance with the pulsatile blood flow. The adventitia consists of mast cells, fibroblasts and collagen which all serve to provide structural integrity to the vessel itself.

Ageing of the aorta leads to changes such as collagen remodelling, calcification, VSMC migration, medial thickening and lumen narrowing [9]. These changes often involve a degree of immunopathology which drives the pathogenesis of the resultant aneurysms. These include pro-inflammatory processes driven by complex interaction between inflammatory cells, cytokines and their respective receptors. In many, these degenerative changes occur at an accelerated rate such that it grossly exceeds the effects of normal ageing and eventually presents itself as an aortic aneurysm.

Aortic aneurysms can occur anywhere along the length of the aorta and can affect the aortic root, aortic arch, thoracic aorta and abdominal aorta. While the underlying immunopathology aspect to their aetiology may be applicable to all, the more common abdominal aorta aneurysm (AAA) is typically associated with atherosclerosis and pro-inflammatory processes.

On the other hand, thoracic aorta aneurysms (TAA) are typically associated with genetically defective connective tissues, medial degeneration and mechanical aetiologies [10]. However, there is now increasing interest in the inflammatory aspects of thoracic aneurysms [2,11]. The differences in aetiology between different aneurysms may be attributed to their inherent structural differences: thoracic aorta containing higher elastic content and more vascular media compared to the avascular abdominal aorta that generally receives greater plaque deposition [12]. Regardless, a myriad of cellular changes and immunological processes can be observed across each type of aneurysm and will be explored in this chapter.

The immunopathology of the various aneurysms can include apoptosis of VSMC, changes to elastin, collagen and glycosaminoglycan (GAG) content, as well as an abundance of reactive oxygen species (ROS) and nitric oxide (NO) [13]. Much of these actions are mediated by the effector cells of both innate and adaptive response. Innate system includes macrophages, neutrophils, natural killer cells, mast cells and dendritic cells whereas the adaptive system include various subtypes of B and T lymphocytes. The innate immune system is traditionally recognised as the chief regulators of inflammation associated with infections and tissue damage whereby dysregulation of its underlying mechanisms leads to prolonged and overzealous immune responses [14]. These actions are mediated by pattern recognition receptors (PRR) such as Toll-like receptors (TLRs) and NOD-like receptors (NLRs), and recognise pathogen-associated molecular pattern (PAMPs) and damage-associated molecular patterns (DAMPs). These have been associated with the development and progression of vascular diseases such as atherosclerosis [15–17]. Furthermore, their activation directly affects the adaptive immune response through direct involvement in the recruitment of antigen-presenting cells, T cells and B cells [18]. The involvement of adaptive system and the subsequent production of various immunoglobulins, cytokines and matrix metalloproteinases are also known to contribute to aneurysm formation through chronic inflammatory changes and signal further changes in cells of the innate system [19,20].

Macrophage

One of the key modulators involved in inflammatory aspect of aneurysm development are macrophages. Their effects are marked by infiltration into the aortic wall and their subsequent roles in extracellular matrix (ECM) degradation, impairment and death of VSMC [21]. These changes would otherwise be absent in health aortas as inflammatory infiltrates are normally absent [6]. The structural instability caused by ECM disruption is an essential component to aneurysm development. Presence of macrophages and their proinflammatory actions disrupt the delicate balance between destructive remodelling and reparative healing through alterations in ECM production. ECM is typically regulated by opposing actions of proteases, such as matrix metalloproteinases (MMPs) which facilitate ECM destruction, and protease inhibitors, such as tissue inhibitors of matrix metalloproteinases (TIMPs). Their roles in AAA pathogenesis have been readily observed, with raised MMPs and deficient inhibitors like TIMPs [22–26]. The ECM degradation will further attract chemotaxis of macrophages to infiltrate and upregulate the inflammatory process, leading to a chronic inflammatory feedback loop [27]. The cytokines released, such as interferon gamma (IFN-γ), in turn impairs ECM production by VSMCs [28]. Despite evidence of their roles, macrophages subtypes have been identified and are now known to vary in function.

Since its discovery in the 19th century, macrophages have received significant attention and is now known to play major roles across various immunological functions [29]. Most macrophages are derived from monocytes that, with the aid of vascular cell adhesion molecules, extravasate out of blood vessels during acute phases of inflammation [30,31]. As they are found in all tissues of the body, they are equipped with the ability to adapt to different environments through polarisation towards M1 or M2 phenotypes. Macrophages typically display CD68 and the M1 and M2 subpopulations differ in the presence of mannose receptor (MR) expression [32]. M1 macrophages, which is MR negative, is traditionally considered as the pro-inflammatory phenotype whereas M2, which is MR positive, is known as its anti-inflammatory counterpart. This paradigm is often regarded as oversimplification of their complex behaviour as many macrophages lie within this continuum [29]. While their main functions include phagocytosis, antigen presentation, and cytokine secretion, they have also been associated with aneurysms.

M1 macrophages are typically regarded as part of our immunity against intracellular pathogens, serving to activate $CD4^+$ T helper cells. M1-like behaviour and phenotypes are induced by Th_1 mediated environments rich in TLR, IFNs and tissue necrosis factor-α (TNF-α) signalling, which drives their proteolytic enzyme secretion and production of pro-inflammatory cytokines such as TNF-α, type I IFN, Interleukin (IL)-1β, IL-6, IL-12, IL-18 and IL-23 [29,33–36]. This facilitates the development of pro-inflammatory microenvironments, inducing the expression of CD68, CD86, MHC II, inducible nitric oxide synthase (iNOS), nicotinamide adenine dinucleotide phosphate (NADPH)-peroxidase and chemokines CXCL9 and CXCL10 [37]. Contrary to actions of M1, M2-like macrophages are marked by their expression of CD64 and CD209, induced in T helper cell type 2 (Th_2) and is associated with mediating extent of immune response. M2 produces anti-inflammatory responses through cytokines such as IL-10 or transforming growth factor-β (TGF-β) which is shown to promote ECM remodelling and tissue repair [37].

Various studies, of both murine and human models, have examined the role of M1 and M2 macrophages in the development of aortic aneurysms. Macrophages are derived from monocytes; in aortic aneurysms the pathogenic macrophages are known to stem from $CCR2^+$ monocytes specifically. Once they extravasate from blood and into sites of inflammation, such as aortic wall under mechanical stress, this monocyte's subgroup undergoes a process of differentiation and polarisation into the various macrophage types. One study identified hypertension and angiotensin as a potential driver for polarisation: Moore et al. increased M2 accumulation in the aorta, likely promoting ECM remodelling and collagen deposition [37,38]. Another study identified the involvement of CD31, an immunoregulatory receptor, which promoted M2 polarisation. However, the study examined murine dissecting aortic aneurysms and may not be wholly applicable to human physiology [30]. Similarly, dampening Notch1 signalling in murine aneurysms were found to attenuate macrophage inflammatory activity in AAA through introducing defects in migration and proliferation, preventing macrophage infiltration into aneurysms [39,40]. In a study by Boytard et al. observing the macrophage in AAA, M1 were present predominantly within the adventitia, where the aortic wall is more degraded, while M2 is found mainly in intraluminal thrombi [32]. This supports the notion that the proinflammatory M1 macrophages take in cellular debris and become foam cells which adds to the oxidative stress and further potentiates the inflammatory state [41,42]. Additionally, elastin-derived peptides (EDP), a product of ECM degradation which is found systemically elevated in AAA patients, causes early mortality and polarises towards M1 subtypes [43,44]. The selective upregulation of M1 by EDP creates a positive feedback loop in which M1 further degrades ECM to release more EDP whereas M2 macrophages remain in lower numbers [32,44]. By affecting the balance of the polarisation, there is therapeutic opportunity in targeting aortic aneurysm formation.

Research into potential therapeutic targets of macrophages and monocytes in AA have also been explored. The renin-angiotensin-aldosterone system is another therapeutic target as angiotensin II induces the production of ROS and proinflammatory chemokines, accelerated atherosclerosis and eventual aneurysm development [45]. Its effects are mediated by macrophage activation and destabilisation of elastin and collagen in the aortic wall, chiefly through C-C chemokine receptor (CCR) 2 which normally regulates monocyte recruitment. CCR^+ monocyte populations differ from CCR^- phenotypes in that they migrate to sites of injury and cause inflammation, rather than becoming resident macrophages and dendritic cells in healthy tissues [46,47]. These potentially pathogenic $CCR2^+$ phenotypes are elevated in both blood and aortic tissue in aneurysms, with an increased number correlated to the degree of aortic dilatation [47]. Similarly, inflammatory monocytes are greatly reduced in mice with CCR2 knocked out [48]. A study that investigated a CCR2 blockade using small interfering RNA achieved substantial inhibition of aneurysm development but, again, its significance is limited by murine models [49]. Immunosuppressants, such as rapamycin inhibitors which affects messenger

RNA production, were used to suppress CCR2 mediated monocyte development as well as reduce aortic dilatation successfully [47]. Suppressive effects of other drugs such as clarithromycin was also able to reduce macrophage infiltration (0.05 versus 0.16; P<0.01) and elastin degradation (56.3% versus 16.5%; P<0.001) [50]. It was also successful at reducing their proinflammatory activities such as release of MMP-2 (P<0.01), MMP-9 (P<0.01), interleukin 1β (346.6 versus 1066.0; P<0.05), IL-6 (128.4 versus 346.2; P<0.05) and overall downregulation of NF-κB (0.3 versus 2.0; P<0.01) [50]. Similarly, inflammatory responses can be attenuated by substituting precursors of proinflammatory cytokines with polyunsaturated fatty acids such as eicosapentaenoic acid (EPA) and docosahexaenoic acid (DHA) [51]. DHA and EPA were shown to significantly suppress both macrophage infiltration and AAA development in mice [52]. Accompanying these changes are a global decrease in the proinflammatory molecules such as TNF-α, TGF-β, MMP-2, MMP-9 and VCAM-1.

Different macrophage subtypes likely contribute differently to aortic remodelling in vascular injury or atherosclerosis. M1 macrophages play dominant roles at the site of injury and lead proinflammatory processes such as cytokine signalling, proteolysis and phagocytosis. Later stages also include M2 macrophages and their involvement in tissue repair processes such as angiogenesis and ECM deposition. It is clear that AAA, rather than TAA, remains under the spotlight as aetiology of TAA is still generally regarded as genetic rather than inflammatory. M1/M2 macrophage ratio also remains a topic of interest to better quantify its role in the development of aortic aneurysm. It is import to note that most evidence of macrophage-oriented therapeutics are murine-based and mostly limited to AAA development; a better understanding in general of their respective roles and interactions in aortic remodelling may eventually lead to new targets in both the management and prevention of aortic aneurysms.

Neutrophils

Similar to monocytes and macrophages, neutrophils, or polymorphonuclear lymphocytes, are also essential to immune responses. They are effector cells that mainly reside in peripheral vasculature and readily migrate into body tissue. While they are best known for phagocytic capabilities, they also actively recruit other effector cells and undergo apoptosis upon phagocytosis [53,54]. Their functions are achieved through various actions: degranulation, formation of neutrophil extracellular traps (NETs) and generation of oxidative bursts [55,56]. While NETs and oxidative bursts are primarily involved in pathogen capture and break down, they work alongside degranulation mechanisms that can lead to proinflammatory behaviours and MMP-mediated ECM remodelling [54,57,58]. The contents of the granules include myeloperoxidase (MPO) and neutrophil elastase (NE) whereas MMP-9 can be found in tertiary granules. MPO, NE and MMP-9 are all heavily involved in matrix degradation and plays a role in aortic aneurysm development.

Although not featured as prominently as monocytes or macrophages, neutrophils are consistently found in aneurysmal aortic walls and is thought to facilitate AA development by initiating the inflammatory response [59,60]. Neutrophils isolated from AAA are found to be activated and more readily releases MPO and oxidative agents such as hydrogen peroxide [61,62]. While exact mechanics of their involvement remains unclear, they are thought to initiate the early inflammatory response from within intramural thrombus, where it recruits other inflammatory cells to produce the signature changes in the aortic wall. They play a role in both the acute inflammatory changes as well as its shift into chronic remodelling, likely through dipeptidyl peptidase I (DPPI). DPPI activates and increases secretion of neutrophil-derived serine proteases such as NE, cathepsin G and proteinase 3 (PR3), which furthers the proinflammatory processes [63–66]. Some of their actions include inducing neutrophil collagenase (MMP-8) and elastases that breaks down the elastin and collagen integral to aortic wall stability [67,68]. Similarly, the neutrophils were also discovered to interact with MMP-2 and MMP-9 by storing and activating them upon their secretion by macrophages. Combined with their tendency to infiltrate the aortic wall, this likely plays an important role in exacerbating wall degradation [69–71]. As a result, increased inflammatory cell infiltration, wall thickening and elastin degradation can be observed. Furthermore, positive feedback response akin to those seen in macrophage activation can be observed in neutrophils because byproducts of elastin fragmentation are potent chemoattractants for neutrophils [72–74].

Many of the above actions by neutrophils increases oxidative stress on the aorta and is thought to cause aortic aneurysms. A study by Kim et al. was able to demonstrate that MPO deficiency can reduce aneurysm incidence and maximum aortic diameter in murine models [75]. Histologically, the aorta walls had significantly less thrombus formation, macrophages and elastase degradation compared to controls. Furthermore, MMP-2 and MMP-9 and serum amyloid A, another indicator of oxidative stress, are also markedly reduced. Similarly, neutrophil proteases and DPPI are found to cause an immediate increase in AAA diameter in mice and that DPPI deficiency significantly suppressed aneurysm formation [67]. Histological analysis of aortic tissue were akin to MPO deficiency, with preservation of elastic lamellae and reduced inflammatory cell infiltrates, especially of macrophages. Additionally, they showed that AAA were significantly smaller in mice with NE or PR3 deficiencies. AAA incidence was also significantly reduced when neutropenia was induced using cytotoxic antibodies in mice ($P<0.001$) [60]. Both tissue neutrophils and macrophages significantly decreased as well ($P=0.005$). This study associated aneurysm suppression with MMP-8 only, rather than MMP-2 or MMP-9, possibly suggesting MMP-8 to be more critical to neutrophil-mediated aneurysm development. Through selectively targeting IL-1β, a neutrophil activator, and ceramides, compounds that stimulate NET activity, AAA protection can be conferred in murine models [58]. By knocking out IL-1β, Meher et al. reduced ceramide production which led to significantly lower neutrophil infiltration of the aortic wall, protecting against AAA development.

Thus far, research has identified many novel therapeutic targets of aortic aneurysms surrounding neutrophils. However, the majority of our knowledge on neutrophil contributions are limited to murine and rodent models. This remains a large barrier as pathophysiology is not always applicable between our species and will require much more investigation in human or primate models. Similarly, the majority of focus rests on AAA, leaving TAAs underexplored.

Mast Cells, Basophils and Eosinophils

The common myeloid progenitor cells that give rise to monocytes and neutrophils also produce mast cells, basophils and eosinophils. Like neutrophils, these are all granulocytes and are best known for their involvement in atopy and immune modulation [76]. They originate from bone marrow and migrate to blood and bodily tissues until appropriate activating signals to trigger further changes. Mast cells and basophils are typically activated by antigen-bound IgE and activated complements, forming the basis of atopy and anaphylaxis. Their activation leads to degranulation of various substances including histamine, serine proteases and proteoglycans as well as powerful inflammatory mediators such as TNF-α, IL-3, IL-5, IL-8 and GM-CSF [76]. Similarly, basophils mainly secrete histamine but differs in the additional expression of potent cytokines IL-4 and IL-13 which serves to influence T helper cell differentiation. Additionally, basophils also produce potent leukotrienes known to increase vascular permeability. Atopy aside, basophils are known to be involved in host defence against parasites. Finally, eosinophils are also involved in allergy and helminth defences and can be activated via IgA and IgG. They degranulate to release highly cytotoxic proteins with anti-helminth activity and is also related to hyperresponsivity. Despite sharing similar effector functions and surface receptors, their exact roles and mechanisms in maintaining immunity and immunopathology remains largely unknown. Their roles in the formation of aortic aneurysms should also be considered as there is literature, albeit limited, that suggest possible associations.

The role of these cells in aneurysm development has gained interests over recent years. Apart from histamine, mast cells also produce tryptase and chymase which degrades ECM via MMP and induces VSMC apoptosis

[77]. This draws an increasing attention towards adventitial mast cells in aneurysms. In 2007, Sun et al. found that mast cells accumulated in murine AAA lesions and that AAA failed to develop in mast cell-deficient mice [78]. These mice experienced reduced amount of aortic expansion, number of macrophages as well as elastic lamina degradation. Similarly, when murine mast cells were artificially activated using degranulation agents, AAA growth can be enhanced. The stabilisation of mast cells was also effective at impeding AAA formation through reducing IL-6 and IFN-γ release, and suggested that they are involved in VSMC apoptosis, matrix protease expression and vascular remodelling. Another study also found raised mast cell numbers in media and adventitia of human AAA, corroborating with previous findings in murine models [77]. They identified correlation between mast cell numbers and diameter of aneurysms as well. The authors also used degranulation inhibitors to isolate the effector role of mast cells and successfully attenuated AAA formation in rodent models. Furthermore, their cell culture revealed mast cells augment the MMP-9 activity originating from macrophages.

Basophils, however, have received little attention but is likely to be involved due to its IL-4 and IL-13 secretion [4]. The two cytokines have a range of functions and includes enhancing B cell proliferation, DC differentiation, T cell proliferation and differentiation. Additionally, it augments production of many cytokines including CCL2 and CCL5 that are produced from EC and VSMC [4]. Additionally, as T lymphocytes are present throughout the development of aortic aneurysms, its potential should be thoroughly explored.

Eosinophils are also under-studied but have been associated TAAs more than AAAs. A study on the role of IgG in inflammatory TAAs found increased eosinophils present in most cases [11]. This was found in the presence of significant thickening of adventitia, elastic fibre damage and lack of calcifying atherosclerotic changes in tunica media. While the study examined 376 patients who underwent TAA surgeries, the observed changes seen may be attributed to the much varied aetiopathogenesis of TAAs which can include atherosclerosis and hypertensive cardiovascular disease to connective tissue disorders and medial degeneration. A case study on owl monkey eosinophilic aortitis and TAA also examined eosinophils. They associated the pathology with autoimmune vasculitides like polyarteritis nodosa, granulomatosis with polyangiitis, eosinophilic granulomatosis with polyangiitis and giant cell arteritis, all of which are characterised by eosinophil infiltration that damages small, medium and occasionally large vessel [79]. There is also evidence to further investigate eosinophil as lower cell count had a slightly increased hazard ratio (1.10; 95% CI 0.62-1.94) [80]. Furthermore, a study by Liu et al. established association between asthma and AAA, presumably sharing common inflammatory mechanics [81].

Dendritic Cells

Dendritic cells (DCs) are central to our immunity through communicating presence of pathogens to direct antigen-specific responses rather than directly destroying pathogens [82]. This bridges the innate and adaptive immune systems and is achieved through careful surveillance and degradation of antigens followed by presentation via MHC I and MHC II. While macrophages and B cells can also present antigens, DCs are exceptionally efficient and is uniquely responsible for antigen-specific responses. By also directly producing cytokines, such as IL-12, they are equipped to activate and stimulate T cell activity. Furthermore, their antigen presentation can also directly stimulate B cells. Additionally, DCs play a regulatory role by maintaining immune tolerance through constant surveillance and presentation of self-antigens to T cells. Such behaviours lead to differentiation of regulatory T cells (Tregs) which downregulates immune responses. DCs exist as distinctive populations that are specialised to the tissues they reside in and can play different immunological roles, including Langerhan cells, plasmacytoid DCs (pDCs) and conventional DCs [82]. Unlike conventional DCs, pDCs are a divergent subset that specialise in targeting viral infections and known to produce large amounts of type I interferons whereas Langerhan cells are DCs that reside in the epidermis [82]. DCs have been observed to be present in atherosclerotic plaques and aortic wall, hence would likely contribute towards the development of aortic aneurysms.

Activated DCs have been known to accumulate in atherosclerotic lesions in aortic tunica intima and throughout the development of aortic aneurysms [47]. This contrasts with the immature phenotypes that are typically found in normal human aortae [83,84]. Their function lies within aortic sclerotic plaques through the 5-lipoxygenase (5-LO) pathway, generating proinflammatory leukotriene lipid mediators [85]. Zhao et al. demonstrated that the 5-LO deficiency attenuates murine aneurysm formation as well as associated it with reduced MMP-2 and macrophage inflammatory protein (MIP)-1α activity. It was identified that one of the downstream products of 5-LO, leukotriene-D4 (LTD$_4$), strongly stimulates the expression of MIP-1α and MIP-2, by macrophages and ECs respectively, which contribute to aortic wall inflammation and aneurysm formation. Atherosclerotic activity was further investigated by Ludewig et al. which associated DC-mediated presentation of atherosclerosis-related antigens with an increase in lesion formation [86]. Their findings reiterate the self-perpetuating nature of the proinflammatory nature of AAAs. Such activities are not limited to conventional DCs but also pDCs which are found within atherosclerotic lesions too [87]. Given that these pDCs are highly responsive to bacterial and viral infections, they may play a role in inflammatory activation in plaques during acute infections [88]. Similarly, DCs are known to reside in tissues such as arterial wall which experience mechanical strain due to blood flow [89]. In murine models, mechanically stressed DCs significantly stimulated T cell proliferation and corresponded with an increased expression of stimulatory and costimulatory molecules on the surface of DC. Unlike conventional DCs and pDCs, DCs of the epidermis called Langerhan cells, are less explored. Only a case study of aortic aneurysm in a patient with giant cell arteritis specifically identified Langerhan cells, which had a prominent presence in aortic wall [90].

As seen, there is plenty of theoretical mechanisms through which DCs can participate in the development of aortic aneurysms but there is a lack of research to examine them specifically. Majority of literature that examine histology only briefly include the presence of DCs and, like many other immunological cells, research remains limited to murine AAA models.

T Lymphocytes

As discussed, involvement of specific antigens have not been thoroughly explored yet and the focus remains on the immunological cells present in the development of aortic aneurysms [91]. Alongside innate immunological cells, T cells are also commonly seen in aneurysmal tissues. Effector T cells stem from the activation of naïve T cells which happens upon presentation of antigen and costimulatory signals by APCs [92]. Effector T cells can be stimulated to differentiate into two broad groups: T helper cells and cytotoxic T cells. Helper cells include T helper type 1 (Th_1), T helper type 2 (Th_2), T helper type 17 (Th_{17}) and regulatory T cells (Tregs) which serve to recruit and activate other cells via cytokines. Other T cells such as $CD8^+$ cytotoxic T cells ($CD8^+$ T cells) aims to eliminate pathogen-infected host cells, as well as natural killer T cells (NKT cells) and γδ T cells which are involved in antipathogen, anti-tumour and autoreactivity regulation [93]. In the presence of intracellular pathogens, cytokines such as IFN-α, IFN-β and IL-12 stimulate differentiation of Th_1, characterised by the persistent release of IFN-γ and TNF-α, serving to upregulate macrophage and APC activities. Similarly, $CD8^+$ T cells are also stimulated by IFN-α, IFN-β and IL-12, serving to recognise and kill infected cells. When stimulated by the IL-4 produced during parasitic responses, Th_2 cells are induced to promote activity of mast cells, basophils and eosinophils via IL-4, IL-5 and IL-13. Differentiation of Th_{17} cells are mediated by cytokines induced by extracellular bacterial or fungal pathogens, such as TGF-β, IL-6, IL-21 and IL-23. The differentiated Th_{17} then stimulates neutrophil recruitment and ROS production via IL-8 and IL-17. With such potent inflammatory potential, modulation of T cell activity and autoimmunity is achieved through Treg and their production of suppressive cytokines such as IL-10, TGF-β and IL-35. After the primary response terminates, the T cell population collapses, leaving a few memory T cells with lower requirements for subsequent activation and an increased proliferative potential. With such diverse functions and cytokine repertoire, much of T cell activities may be implicated, either directly or indirectly, in the development of aortic aneurysms. In particular, their stimulatory effects on innate immune system like macrophages and neutrophils warrants attention.

T helper cells are cellular infiltrates commonly found in AAAs and has been implicated in the pathophysiology. Xiong et al. used $CaCl_2$-induced aneurysm murine models to demonstrate the lack of response in T cell deficient mice [94]. On histological examination, aortic tissue had no T cell infiltration either, further demonstrating their involvement in AAA development. Similarly, the primary Th_1 cytokine, IFN-γ, was also implicated. Aneurysm development in IFN-γ-deficient mice were suppressed and revealed similar elastic lamellae to control groups. These changes were also associated with significantly less T cell infiltration and the subsequent reduction of MMP-2 and MMP-9. Th_2 have also been implicated in IgG4-related AA through its use of cytokines such as IL-4, IL-10 and IL-13 [95]. Both serum IL-10 and IL-13 were upregulated and significantly higher in IgG4-AA than both the normal aorta as well as non-IgG4-related AAs. As IL-10 and IL-13 promote Ig production towards IgG4, Kasashima et al. concluded that it reflected the involvement of Th_2 and Tregs on AA development in the setting of IgG4-related diseases. The role of various T cells remains to be substantiated as contradicting evidence have been seen. King et al. found that IFN-γ secretion by Th_1 attenuated AAA development instead, and its deficiency associated with increased aneurysmal rupture mortality ($P<0.05$) [96]. Similarly, these findings were agreed by Shimizu et al. whose IFN-γ blockade increased murine AAA severity along with raised MMP-2 and MMP-9 expression [97]. Th_{17} cells, and its signature cytokine IL-17, have also been implicated in AAA development. They are both upregulated in aortic dissection patients, associated with onset of AD in humans [98]. Furthermore, through antagonising Th_{17} differentiation with digoxin, Th_{17} and IL-17 related inflammatory processes in murine AAA models were successfully attenuated in a dose-dependent manner [99].

Smaller T cell subsets such as CD8⁺ cytotoxic T cells, NKT and γδ cells have not been studied as often. There is some evidence to implicate CD8⁺ T cells in promoting aneurysm formation. They may make up to 50% of the T cell infiltrates in atherosclerotic plaques and is thought to target macrophages, VSMCs and ECs for apoptosis [100]. Another study associated IFN-γ producing CD8⁺ T cells, but not CD4⁺ T cells, with AA development via apoptosis and MMP activity levels [101]. NKT cells were also identified in atherosclerotic plaques within human AAA lesions and thought to aggravate AAA development [102,103]. The presence of NKT cells allows interaction with Th$_1$ which is thought to destabilise AAA through inhibition of VSMC proliferation and induction of apoptosis [104]. NKT cells are also known to secrete IL-4 which may contribute through increasing MMP expression of VSMC and macrophages [105]. Similarly, γδ cells were implicated when found clonally expanded in AAA lesions in multiple studies [106,107]. Zhang et al. found that AAA formation was significantly attenuated in γδ knockout mice and saw an associated upregulation of proliferation-related genes, such as *Mtor* and *Myc*. A reciprocal downregulation of apoptosis related genes, such as *Bcl1* and *Bad* was also noted [108]. Their results suggested that γδ T cells may be involved in AA development through cell proliferation and regulation of inflammatory responses. While investigation into memory T cells is limited, infiltrating CD4⁺ and CD8⁺ T cells in AAA lesions have been shown to be a uniquely activated memory phenotype [109,110]. This was accompanied with the chemokine receptor profile of a predominantly type 1 mediated response against the aortic wall. The presence of these activated memory cells is likely to contribute through their ability to produce high amounts of inflammatory cytokines such as IFN-γ and IL-2 [111].

Without the inhibitory effect of Tregs on T cells, aneurysms are also more likely to form. In a study by Ait-Oufella et al., depletion of Tregs via the use of CD25 antibodies significantly enhances susceptibility of mice to AAA and aortic rupture (P=0.009) [112]. Similar results were achieved in mice with impaired Treg homeostasis. Treg depletion was associated with a loss of IL-10 anti-inflammatory response leading to an increased immune cell activation. Restoration of Tregs in Treg-deficient mice restores the immunoinflammatory balance, preventing the development of AAA and dissection. This is reiterated by Ohkura et al. who identified a significant AAA mortality in Treg deficiency [59,113]. Furthermore, Tregs are shown to be protective of AAA progression through the release of TGF-β, a powerful Th_1 and Th_2 differentiation regulator [114]. Wang et al. showed that the deficiency of TGF-β was associated with VSMC death, elastin degradation and increased vascular inflammatory response. Similar to the effects of other T cells, there is contrasting evidence for the involvement of TGF-β that will be further discussed [115].

In short, T cells are of a diverse group and has been implicated in the development of aortic aneurysms. However, current knowledge on TAA is lacking and remains centred around AAA. There is also conflicting literature on both the effects and mechanism of how these cells partake in the pathophysiology. While likely to harbour therapeutic potential, this area needs further clinical investigation to substantiate and consolidate our current knowledge.

B Lymphocytes

B cells are responsible for both humoral and cellular immunity, achieved through antibody production as well as T cell activation via antigen presentation [116]. B cells are generally classified into B1 and B2, which is further subdivided into marginal zone (MZ) and follicular (FO) B cells. B1 cells secrete IgA as well as IgM, which has been implicated in recognising altered self-antigens by apoptotic cells in injured tissues [117]. Similarly, MZ B cells serve to secrete IgM and clear apoptotic cells. Both cells are equipped with TLRs to recognise PAMPs and endogenous ligands, independent of antigen recognition via BCR, allowing for rapid IgM mediated responses during infections. FO B cells, however, make up the majority of the B cell lineages, residing in secondary lymphoid tissues such as spleen and lymph nodes. They provide long-lasting humoral immunity mediated by IgG and is activated with the help of T cells. Most B cells arise from bone marrow, except B1 which originates from foetal liver, and are released into the bloodstream as immature B cells. As they mature, gene segments of immunoglobulin are rearranged to produce unique B cell receptors and allow further differentiation into plasma cells and memory B cells upon exposure to foreign antigens. Presence of B cells infiltrates in aortic walls and the production of immunoglobulins, IgG4 in particular, have been associated with AA development and warrants attention.

While T cells are the predominant lymphocyte in AAA, B cells have also been implicated in AA development. Within these AAA lesions, B cells have been observed to form lymphoid follicles with germative centres, infiltrated by T cells and DCs. This suggests that antigen presentation may happen directly within the aortic wall [118]. Meher et al. found B2 cells to be the predominant subset in AAA lesions of mice [119]. This was coupled with an increase in splenic Treg population and the suppression of AAA formation. The use of rituximab, a B cell depleting drug targeting CD20 on B cells, have also been used in mice AAA [120]. Schaheen et al. successfully depleted both B1 and B2 population and suppressed AAA growth (control versus anti-CD20; 97.9±7.4% versus 62.2±4.7%; P<0.01) [120]. Results of the study were accompanied by lowered IgM levels (P<0.01), contradicting the findings of DiLillo et al. where IgM levels remained similar between depletion and control groups [121].

Various immunoglobulin products from plasma cells have received attention in the setting of aortic aneurysms. Inflammatory AA is characterised by high serum IgG4 and IgE levels, thought to be a systemic vascular disease [122]. IgG4, for example, is the least abundant IgG but most commonly associated with inflammatory AAs were IgG4$^+$ plasma cells in the aortic wall of AAA, contributing to aortic dilation [59,123,124]. This involvement becomes more apparent as B cell depletion therapy has been shown to be protective AAA [120]. However, this study also found no changes to level of IgG, cytokines or chemokines. Similarly IgE in high concentration is thought to also promote atherosclerosis and dilation [125–128]. This is particularly apparent in AAA formation in those with higher IgE such as hyper-IgE syndrome. The role of IgE likely is not limited to interaction with mast cells, eosinophils and basophils but also extends to the activation of T cells and macrophages [129]. Alternatively, IgM is positively correlated with inflammatory disease, found in the adventitia of AAA [130,131]. IgM secretion models interestingly show its facilitation of atherosclerosis while natural IgM production by B1 cells have shown to be protective [127,132,133].

B cells and immunoglobulins have been demonstrated to be injurious in various murine AAA models but is often limited by contradictory findings as well as lack of attention on specifically TAA or FO or MZ B cells. Despite the therapeutic potential of B cell depletion having already been explored and implemented in various autoimmune and oncological diseases, the lack of specific studies on human AA remains a barrier.

Innate Lymphoid Cells

Last group of lymphocytes to be discussed is innate lymphoid cells (ILCs), which includes a variety of cells with similar functions and phenotype as lymphocytes but lacks the signature rearranged receptors of adaptive immune cells [134]. A key characteristic is that they do not express classical B cell, T cell or myeloid surface receptors. They can be classified in various ways but most commonly divided into subgroups of ILC1, ILC2 and ILC3. ILC1, which notably includes natural killer (NK) cells, is characterised by IFN-γ production and cytotoxic activities [135]. ILC2 are marked by their production of Th_2-like cytokines such as IL-5 and IL-13 whereas ILC3 is known for Th_{17}-like activities through IL-17 and IL-22 secretion [136]. All three ILC categories are developed through IL-7 exposure, with the exception of IL-15 specifically required for NK cell differentiation. These cells play a similar role as effector T cells and may also contribute towards aneurysm development.

Attention directed towards ILCs have gradually increased in recent years, and is now studied in the context of vascular disease and pathogenesis. NK cells are among the cells most commonly found in aortic wall infiltrate in AAAs and is associated with plaque formation, atherosclerosis and vascular damage through various studies [137]. In 1997, Seko et al. demonstrated for the first time that perforin-expressing NK cells directly injure or kill vascular cells in human AAA. Following this, AAA patients were identified to have significantly more NK cells than controls (23.8 versus 16.2; P<0.01), showing increased cytotoxic activity towards VSMC [138]. Certain NK cells subsets have also been associated with destabilisation of carotid plaques in a human study [139]. Similarly, depletion of NK cells alone in murine models was found to significantly attenuate atherosclerosis and that the transferral of NK cells confirms an atherogenic role [140]. Despite displaying similar activity profiles to various T cell phenotypes, ILCs have generally been ignored in aortic aneurysms. However, ILC2 and IL-33 signalling pathway have been implicated in AAA in a recent study [141]. IL-33 is a cytokine released from damaged or necrotic cells and can activate IL-33 receptors on Th_1, Th_2, Treg and ILC2 and is thought to regulate local immune response. The study found IL-33 protective against AAA development, in concordance of the fact that ILC2 activated by IL-33 will induce Treg accumulation, which is known to confer protection [142]. Finally, ILC2 have also been found in para-aortic adipose tissue and ablation of this population in mice accelerated atherosclerotic development. This removes the atheroprotective immunity mediated by ILC2 production of IL-5 and IL-13 and is in concordance with similar protective effects seen in the previous study [143].

While attention on ILCs are rising, the majority have been focused on NK and ILC2. Similar to many other cells, literature is wholly limited to AAA and mostly murine models. Given the likeness of their activity with T cells, ILCs remain a target for further research to fully explore their therapeutic potential.

Toll-Like and NOD-Like Receptors

Toll-like receptors (TLR) and nucleotide-binding and oligomerisation domain-like receptors (NLR), or NOD-like receptors, are PRR discovered in the 1990s. They are cellular detectors of PAMPs and DAMPs, modulating cellular activation, proliferation and apoptotic activities. Located on 4q31.3, the TLR gene has five exons and is typically expressed in the appendix and bone marrow [144]. Of the thirteen different TLR receptors, TLR2 was identified along with TLR1, TLR3, TLR4, TLR5. They trigger an immune response upon recognition of PAMP such as cell membrane, cell wall and bacterial toxins [145]. TLRs are type 1 integral membrane glycoproteins. Its N-terminal has leucine-rich repeats and the C-terminal is the Toll/IL-1 receptor (TIR). TLR2 binds to a great diversity of microbial ligands including Diacyl lipopeptides from Mycoplasma, heat-labile enterotoxins from Escherichia coli and Vibrio cholerae, and peptidoglycan from Staphylococcus. After TLR2 binds to its ligand, it triggers a signalling pathway through TLR1 or TLR6 to achieve adaptive immunity. NLR, on the other hand, are categorised by its N-terminal domain, into NLRA, NLRB, NLRC and NLRP, typically expressed in immune cells and epithelial cells [146]. They are involved in inflammasome assembly, signalling transduction, transcription activation and autophagy [147]. As NLR polymorphisms have also been associated with autoimmune diseases such as Crohn disease, it is possible that similar mechanics may contribute to AA development [145].

Currently, the actions and implications of TLRs and NLRs have had some attention in the setting of AA development. Lai et al. suggested that TLR4 is essential for the development of AAA [148]. A murine $CaCl_2$-induced AAA model was used, with observations of TLR4 on day 3 post-exposure and reaching its peak on day 14. Evaluation of AAA formation in TLR4-deficient mice was shown to be significantly lower in knockout mice. Aortic diameter was significantly smaller (0.60±0.03 mm versus 0.90±0.04 mm; $P<0.001$) along with lower expression of TNF-α, IL-6, MCP-1 and MMPs. Similarly, in the setting of sporadic TAA, Pisano et al. suggested a model of the role of TLR4 in pathophysiology [2]. As TLR4 is widely expressed in EC and VSMC, activation of TLR4 by DAMPs lead to endothelial dysfunction, changes in vascular tone, degradation of ECM and elastin fragmentation. However, it is important to note that the level of cytokines did not correlate with aneurysm size. Alternatively, commonly used drugs such as antimalarials, angiotensin receptor blockers, and statins have been found to affect immune responses. They are regarded as small molecule inhibitors, acting through the modulation of intravesical pH as well as affecting endosomal TLR signalling [149]. Similarly, molecules like lipid A antibodies and oligonucleotides are found to prevent ligand receptor binding as well as certain microRNAs that can inhibit the intracellular signalling cascade of the TLR pathway. Exploration of these molecules may open up novel TLR targeting therapeutics in AA as it is already implemented in autoimmune diseases such as arthritis and systemic lupus erythematosus.

Certain NLR alleles have received particular attention; Wu et al. examined the role of NLRP3 caspase-1 inflammasome in VSMC contractile dysfunction in AA and AD. A significant amount of degradation of aortic VSMC contractile protein was observed in patients with sporadic thoracic AA ($P<0.0001$) [150]. This was associated with the activation of the NLRP3 caspase-1 inflammasome cascade. Mice that are NLRP3 or caspase-1 inflammasome deficient showed reduced angiotensin II-induced protein degradation and increased biochemical dysfunction and aneurysm formation. This is seen by the significant increase in AA and AD ($P<0.05$). Similarly, Roberts et al. assessed the association between NLRP3, CARD8 and AAA [151]. 1151 patients with AAA and 727 controls were genotyped and frequency of the various alleles are recorded. The results showed that CARD8 provided a protective effect against AAA when applying a recessive genetic model (OR=0.83; P=0.047; 95% CI 0.69-0.99). When pairing the two genotypes, the CARD8/NLRP3 pair conferred a protective effect over other combinations. However, contrasting the study by Wu et al., NLRP3 showed no association with overall disease and susceptibility of AAA development.

Human Leukocyte Antigen

Human specific major histocompatibility complex (MHC) is known as human leukocyte antigen (HLA). It is a polymorphic gene located on the 6p21 loci, encoding α chains of MHC I and both α and β chains of MHC Class II [152]. Responsible for antigen presentation, MHC are clinically important in maintaining self-tolerance and for recognition of foreign antigens. They function through initiating T cell responses and subsequent activation of other downstream immune effectors through binding of various self and foreign antigens. Their importance can be exemplified by the need for full HLA assessments prior to transplants to prevent mismatches and rejections [153]. HLA polymorphisms have also been associated with autoimmune diseases such as diabetes, ankylosing spondylitis and rheumatoid arthritis [154–156]. Despite having a multifaceted aetiology behind aortic aneurysms, the widespread participation of immune cells suggests at least a component of immune dysregulation involved, in which HLA may contribute towards.

A study by Monux et al. suggested that HLA has a role in the formation of AAA by autoimmune processes [157]. 72 patients with AAA and 380 control subjects had HLA typing. 11 alleles of HLA-DRB1 locus were typed. The alleles were identified using oligonucleotide probe and showed the allele subtype HLA-DRB1*0401 to be more common than the AAA group (12.5 versus 5.2%; P=0.02; OR 2.59) [157]. The authors remarked that HLA-DRB1*0401 is associated to severe form of rheumatoid arthritis but it does not mean it is responsible for the development of the disease. Therefore more research is needed to determine the effect of HLA-DRB1*0401 on the pathophysiology of AAA. A recent case-control study by Anaya-Ayala et al. showed the association between alleles HLA-DRB1*01, HLA-DR B1*16 and AAA [158]. The study recruited 51 patients with AAA and 99 disease free patients. A total of 102 Class II HLA-DRB1 alleles of AAA patients and 198 from controlled group were analysed. HLA-DRB1*01 had a higher allele frequency in AAA patients compared to control groups (0.139 versus 0.05; P=0.015; OR 3; 95% CI 1.29-7.08). HLA-DR B1*16 also has a higher allele frequency in AAA patients (0.109 versus 0.025; P=0.006; OR 4.7; 95% CI 1.59-13.98). Similarly, a case control study by Ogata et al. looked for potential associations between the HLA-DQA locus and AAA in Belgium and Canadian population [159]. Alleles were determined in 387 cases and 426 controls using PCR. The HLA-DQA1*0102 allele in AAA cases was more common in Belgian males (20.8% versus 12.4%; P=0.003). This allele was found to be protective against autoimmune diseases such as diabetes mellitus and systemic lupus erythematous in other literature [160,161]. However, it is important to note that the use of two populations reduced population stratification, introducing the possibility of a false positive results. Finally, a prospective observational study by Haveman et al. looked at the expression of HLA-DR on monocytes and systemic inflammation in 30 patients with ruptured AAA [162]. Blood samples were taken and the level of CD-14 positive monocytes expressing HLA-DR and IL-6 was measured. Its expression is significantly lower in non-survivors post day 3 ($P<0.05$), suggesting some level of involvement or possible prognostic determination.

Although the exact biological mechanism of HLA on AAA remains unclear, the highlight of genetic and molecular association of AAA may eventually allow for better risk prediction and lower threshold for interventions. This may eventually improve prognosis of aneurysms as the underlying effects of HLA impairment become more apparent.

Immunoregulators

Regulation of inflammatory response are equally important to prevent excessive damage on host tissues. In humans, the T cell activities are controlled through cytotoxic T lymphocyte-associated antigen 4 (CTLA-4) and programmed cell death protein 1 (PD-1). CTLA-4 is expressed on T cells, more specifically $CD4^+$ subsets, and its co stimulatory relationship with CD80 and CD86, membrane proteins of the immunoglobulin superfamily, is arguably the most well researched pathway. It is currently known that activation of CTLA-4 inhibits T cell activity through downregulation of proliferation and expression of various cytokines [163]. Its presence in the blood plasma takes a soluble form likely originated from receptor shedding of cell membranes, a component now known to help identify cellular or biochemical abnormalities [164]. PD-1 and its ligand, programmed death ligand 1 (PD-L1), are more specific, with receptor expressed only on activated T cells and ligands present on macrophages and dendritic cells. Both act as immune checkpoints, co-inhibiting factors and cytokines to limit T cell response; deficiencies lead to failure in regulation of the immune system resulting in overstimulation while excess leads to lost

T cell immunity [165]. When PD-L1 engages PD-1, T cell receptor and CD28 activation cascades, a co-stimulant for T cell survival and proliferation, are decreased. Thus, T cell activation is weakened to reduce strength of immune response [165]. Given the vast involvement and overwhelmingly pro-inflammatory state predisposes AAs, impaired immune regulators will affect and exacerbate the underlying pathophysiology.

A notable decrease of soluble CTLA-4 has been observed in AAA (P=0.0018) and larger aneurysms (P=0.0001) compared to control [166]. Hypertension has also been associated with lowered soluble CTLA-4 (P=0.0002) and a negative correlation has been established between the production of MMP9 and amount of sCTLA-4 (P=0.0006; r=-0.34) [166]. This suggests a viable pathway to connect vascular disease to lowered soluble CTLA-4 is through MMP-9, a well-known proinflammatory cytokine promoting medial degeneration. An increased sCTLA-4 has not been seen to affect aortic vasculature but instead presents a range of other conditions such as systemic lupus erythematosus, asthma and myasthenia gravis [167–169]. Needless to say, those healthy rarely find sCTLA-4 in the plasma [170]. As a co-inhibitory molecule for T cells, the specific details of CTLA-4 function have not been discovered yet. It is known that overexpression reduces AAA incidence (66%) and mortality (26%) in high cholesterol diet murine models; this is accompanied with a notable decrease in $CD4^+$ numbers as well as expression of CTLA ligands, CD80 and CD86 [92]. Although the CTLA-4 overexpression mechanism has yet to be identified with a role in AAA, said role is not associated with the Treg response, a pathway utilising IL-10 anti-inflammatory cytokines to reduce AAA [92]. As a therapeutic target, the anti-CTLA-4 antibody treatment has been effectively used for rheumatoid arthritis, a condition partially linked to atherosclerosis and AAA [171–173]. While often used as autoimmune or cancer treatment, there have been unintended, but remarkable, decreases in CVD in rheumatoid arthritis patients with diabetes mellitus [174]. Thus, it will likely have clinical implications in the prevention, and possibly solution, of CVD-like aetiologies behind AA development.

Similarly, when found on activated T cells and B cells, the expression of both PD-1 and PD-L1 have been found higher in atherosclerotic patients than controls [165]. In coronary artery diseases PDL1 overexpression involves suppression of CD4$^+$ cells while in the formation of atherosclerotic plaque PD-L1 macrophages produces IL-1β and IL-6 anti-inflammatory cytokines to reduce adaptive and increase innate immune response. Giant cell arteritis is another form of vasculitis damage, different from aneurysms, where a lack of PD-L1 attenuated T cell response and loss of PD-1 signals lead to fulminant vasculitis, atherogenesis and increased macrophage and T cell [175,176]. With evidence of PD-1/PD-L1 being problematic when either over- or under-expressed, more investigations are needed to identify its therapeutic potentials.

More research in both CTLA-4 and PD-1/PD-L1 with regards to their roles in aneurysm formation is essential to substantiate the full extent of their clinical implications. We can infer both as viable therapeutic targets based on currently available immunotherapy but specific applications in AA is yet to be known. Again, much of the available literature neglects TAAs and should be investigated thoroughly as well.

Cytokines: IFN-γ, TNF-α, TGF-β1

IFN-γ is an activator of macrophages as part of both the innate and adaptive response. Along with many interleukins, IFN-γ is secreted by NK and CD4 Th$_1$ cells, both of which are cells predominantly found in AAA [177,178]. Much controversy exists with regards to the role of IFN-γ in AAA. Some studies suggest IFN-γ to attenuate AAA formation and development, with evidence of IFN-γ blockades promoting elastic laminae degradation and MMP-9 and -12 formation [97]. Others conclude contradictorily that IFN-γ promotes AAA formation, while deletion attenuates MMP expression and inhibited aneurysm development [94].

On the other hand, TNF-α has a clear role in AAA. Produced by activated macrophages, TNF-α acts as a proinflammatory cytokine alongside IL-1β to promote aneurysm formation, with an increased expression in AAA blood plasma [179–181]. Deletion prevents aneurysm formation, deficiency stunts macrophage recruitment and reduces MMP-2 and -9 expression while antagonists stop elastic fibre disruptions and subsequently aneurysm growth [179]. A study by Xiong et al. showed TNF-α deficiency provide significant protection from murine AAA development, where all 11 mice developed AAA compared to only 2 of 17 in TNF-α knockout mice (P<0.0001). IL-1β and TNF-α are seen hand in hand as the some of the most important proinflammatory factors amongst a variety of diseases including rheumatoid arthritis and inflammatory bowel diseases [181]. Yet TNF-α blockade and antagonists prove more clinically effective than IL-1β targeted treatments. In fact, IL-1β deletion had no significant effect on aneurysm formations and MMP expression [182–184]. Thus, it is likely that interventions based on TNF-α would be effective at treating aortic aneurysms.

TGF-β is responsible for maintenance and development of organs and vasculature, secreted as a complex of cytokines, peptides and latent TGF binding proteins. There is an increase in inactive TGF-β in aortic aneurysms, inferred by an increase in TGF-β mediators such as pSmad2. Some research suggests that a loss of TGF-β reduces dilation and increases risk of aneurysms while others suggest a protective role against aortopathies, ruptures and aneurysm growth [114,185,186]. However, the predominant relationship between TGF-β and aortic aneurysms lies with the genetic mutations involving its signalling pathways [187]. Known to affect matrix degradation and vascular modelling, TGF-β plays a direct role in the development of cardiovascular diseases of Marfan syndrome and Loey-Dietz syndrome amongst others [188–190]. Both these diseases are exhibit hallmark impairment of TGF-β signalling pathways [187,191]. Some studies identify the TGF-β present in such diseases to be mutated variants, playing a causal role through the effects placed on signalling proteins such as fibrillin-1 while mutations in the TGF-β receptors may similarly lead to TAA [187,188,192].

Take TGF-β1 as an example, promoting TAA development and medial degeneration through MMPs [193,194]. Mutations leading to increased TGF-β will further aortic aneurysms, however complete neutralisation of TGF-β similarly causes fatal aortic dissection [114]. That being said, observations of TGF-β signalling in association with aortic aneurysms has yet to produce direct evidence supporting TGF-β's causal role in aneurysm formation [189,195]. The extensive presence of TGF-β may be attributable as a homeostatic response to aortic damage, rendering its role effective instead of causal. Murine models have shown TGF-β to protect against aortic aneurysm progression in early stages of Marfan syndrome, an observation that may be extended to humans [114,196]. Other studies, such as one by Theruvath et al. found TGF-β to downregulate MMP and upregulate MMP inhibitors such as TIMP [197].

Therefore, therapeutic targeting of TGF-β must be carried out carefully considering the complexity of consequences when alterations are made and more research will certainly help achieve better outcomes.

Matrix Metalloproteinases

When we consider the chemokines involved in aortic aneurysms, MMPs predominantly comes to mind. 28 endopeptidase proteins known as matrix metalloproteinases (MMPs) are proteinases that serve to cleave and degrade ECM. They are regulated by TIMPs and MMP antagonists, and plays various roles, from physiological angiogenesis to pathological involvement in cancer and CVD [198–200]. TIMP1, expressed by aortic VSMCs, is found to inhibit most MMPs; MMP-9 in particular [201]. However, the ratio of MMP:TIMP is much higher in AAA than in controls (0.135 versus 0.045; $P=0.018$), suggesting decreased downregulation of MMPs in aneurysm formation [202]. Various MMPs, including -1, -2, -3, -9, -12, -13 and -14, are seen across both TAAs and AAAs. MMP-1, -2 and -9 were found significantly increased in AAA: MMP-2 (27.3±6.3 versus 2.7±0.8 pg MMP-2/μg RNA; $P<0.05$) and MMP-9 (5.9±2.3 vs 0.04±0.01 pg MMP-9/μg RNA). MMP-2 and -9 functioning as gelatinase that degrades denatured fibrillar collagen, elastin and other ECM components [203–205]. MMP-2 and -9 have also been suggested to proteolytically cleave latent TGF-β, a crucial part of the activation process for the potentially proinflammatory molecule [206]. While both play key roles in aneurysm formation, their origins vary [203]. MMP-2 is derived from VSMCs and fibroblasts while

MMP-9 from macrophages and neutrophils; both have multicellular origins making it difficult to target cells in therapeutics [207,208]. That being said, the role of MMP-2 remains unsubstantiated as there is evidence suggesting promotion of thoracic aorta remodelling and others suggesting roles in early aneurysm formation only [209,210]. Others such as MMP-3, is promoted by interleukins and TNF-α, and contributes to plaque destabilisation and elastic lamina degradation [211]. Similarly, production of MMP-12 is stimulated by IL-3 from lymphocytes and VSMCs, a proteinase that co-localises with broken down elastic fibre fragments, furthering aortic aneurysm development [24,212,213].

Oxidants

Within the setting of aneurysm development, various oxidative agents are also known to be involved, chiefly concerning ROS and nitric oxide. ROS is the collection of oxygen derived molecules released by lymphocytes and macrophages [214,215]. NO is a free radical which plays a role in vasodilation, blood flow and cell signalling. ROS and NO are produced by inducible nitric oxide synthase (iNOS) and NADPH oxidases, and serves similar pathogenic roles in aortic aneurysm formation. ROS targets signalling molecules and cell pathways in vascular wall, inducing ECM degradation and vascular dysfunction. Outside of the aorta, ROS affects transcription factors, calcium transport system and more, causing oxidative damage through various mechanisms [214,216]. Impairing vasodilation and cell growth increases risk of AAA, while apoptosis and anoikis, another apoptosis-like process with ECM detachment, plays roles in vascular wall degradation. The activation of adhesion and inflammatory molecules contributes to AAA formation and enhances enzymes inducing ROS production [214]. A positive feedback loop is seen when proinflammatory cytokines, such as IL-1β, TNF-α or IFN-γ, upregulate ROS production in vascular cells via enzymes, such as iNOS and NADPH, leading to further inflammation and apoptosis of aortic vasculature. Studies inhibiting inducible NOS and NADPH reduced ROS, forming direct correlations with the inhibition of matrix degradation and aneurysm formation. Another inflammatory chemokine activated by ROS are MMPs, of which MMP-2 and MMP-9 have been heavily associated with AAA [214,217,218]. Although no direct evidence of ROS effect on aortic aneurysm has been identified, many associations have been made with regards to chronic inflammation, atherosclerosis and AAA [214]. The presence of iNOS in AAA is supported indirectly by many studies but none in human beings thus far. Murine models have been the primary target of research. Studies have confirmed iNOS in association with AAA, for example one study by Zhang J et al. finding 25 of 25 AAA patients with iNOS and virtually no iNOS in the 10 control [219]. Infusion of iNOS enhanced NO production ($P<0.05$) and reduced aneurysm size ($P<0.01$) [220]. Inhibition of iNOS has also been seen to inhibit MMP-13 production, possibly through the role of NO in inducing MMP-13 [221]. In fact, iNOS has been found to play a causal role in AAA development, affecting MMP-2 and -9 activation and expression as well [214]. Some suggest NO induces EMMPRIN, an extracellular MMP inducer, which regulates MMP-13 cleaving of ECM and furthering AAA development [221].

The lipid oxidation hypothesis, a relatively new concept, is suspected in playing a pathological role in AAA via coagulation regulation and vascular inflammation. Enzymatically oxidised phospholipids (eoxPLs) and oxidised phospholipids are both found in murine and human aortic aneurysms tissue, where their deletion reduces AAA severity [222]. The suspected role it plays involves eoxPL deposition on vessel walls, allowing coagulants to bind and activate. Through genetically altered murine models, eoxPL has been found to actively promote AAA via upregulation of IL-6. It has also been found that eoxPL serves different functions and roles in AAA development depending on delivery and location.

Complements

The complement family have always played a role in immunology and the immune component of aortic aneurysms is no different. Autoimmunity of the aorta is prevalent in AAA, particularly through the lectin and classical pathway. C2, the intersection of classical and lectin pathways, is increased in AAA while mRNA of classical proteins, such as C1QA and C1QC, are also elevated [223]. ELISA testing of human AAA patient aortic tissue extract has indicated a 125 fold increase in C3 compared to normal while western blotting found a remnants of degraded complement [224]. Immunoglobulin gamma found in the affected aorta showed even greater increases, such as a 389 fold in IgG3, which may have played an important role if classical pathway activation. Decreased gene expression of complement inhibitors in each pathway has been noted, particularly *CFH*, *SERPING1* and *CD59* in the alternative pathway, classical pathway and membrane attack complex formation respectively [223]. In the elastase induced AAA model, a complete complement depletion protected mice from AAA development [225]. In fact, even the antagonism of C3a alone has been observed to stop AAA development completely. Nonetheless, there exists contradicting studies and questions the observed associations between the complement cascade and AAA [226].

Glycosaminoglycans

Chemokines and cytokines aside, a lesser known molecule named glycosaminoglycan (GAG), plays a selective role in TAA. GAG pooling is the accumulation of glycosaminoglycans, a phenomenon seen in the TAA patients alone [227]. Under normal circumstances, GAGs are polysaccharides that help form parts of the ECM, helping attract water via sodium ion attraction as well as trapping and storing growth factors. Pathologically, the accumulation of GAGs increases risk of delamination and rupture via alteration of aortic pressure and lamina structure. GAGs are negatively charged molecules and they play a compressive role rather than tensile role in the aorta. First, it introduces interstitial water which provides the pressure to separate the lamellae from the aortic wall, as demonstrated by Lesauskaite et al. [228,229]. Second, the presence of GAGs displace other structural components of ECM such as elastic fibres, collagen, and

VSMC, reducing tensile carrying capacity [229]. Third, GAG pooling rarely occurs in a uniform fashion along the aorta but instead deposits in high concentrations at certain regions known as focal stress concentration; this increases local pressure by folds [227,229,230]. Unsurprisingly, chemokines and cytokines affect GAG expression was observed, having found GAG pooling co-localised with MMP-3 and MMP-7 activities, as well as increased GAG production in association with TGF-β activity [231,232]. Albeit a common histopathology, the cause of GAG pooling remains unknown and yet to be explored in detail by current literature [227,228,230,233].

CONCLUSION

This chapter has reviewed various aspects of the pathophysiology behind aortic aneurysms. Development of aneurysms are the resultant product of complex interplay between various cellular, receptor and cytokine components, each contributing to the self-perpetuating inflammatory processes. Key effector cells, such as macrophages and T lymphocytes, have been well explored, along with lesser investigated cells, to demonstrate the widespread changes that underlie the pathophysiology. The mechanics of these cellular actions are being slowly unravelled through parallel research on various cytokines, receptors and effector molecules. These lead to autoimmune-like actions by both innate and adaptive system, ultimately causing damage and destabilisation of aortic wall integrity.

The recognition of immunobiology and pathophysiology behind aortic aneurysms remains rapidly progressing and provide us with evermore potential treatment targets to halt and eventually prevent aneurysm development. Continual exploration of this field will open up better interventions, lower aneurysm ruptures and improve prognosis. However, as much of our knowledge remains limited to abdominal aortic aneurysms in murine models, we are far from maximising their clinical potentials. It is clear that the atherosclerotic aetiology has been well investigated, but we must continue to unravel the sophisticated immunological changes that underlie every aspect of aortic aneurysms.

REFERENCES

[1] Kanasi E, Ayilavarapu S, Jones J. The aging population: demographics and the biology of aging. Vol. 72, *Periodontology 2000*. Blackwell Munksgaard; 2016. p. 13–8.

[2] Pisano C, Balistreri CR, Ricasoli A, Ruvolo G. Cardiovascular disease in ageing: An overview on thoracic aortic aneurysm as an emerging inflammatory disease. Vol. 2017, *Mediators of Inflammation*. Hindawi Limited; 2017.

[3] Lakatta EG, Levy D. Arterial and Cardiac Aging: Major Shareholders in Cardiovascular Disease Enterprises Part I: Aging Arteries: A "Set Up" for *Vascular Disease The Demographic Imperative and the Risk of Vascular Diseases in Older Persons*. Circulation [Internet]. 2003;107(1):139–46. Available from: http://www.circulationaha.org

[4] Shimizu K, Mitchell RN, Libby P. *Inflammation and Cellular Immune Responses in Abdominal Aortic Aneurysms* [Internet]. May, 2006. Available from: http://www.ncbi.nlm.nih.gov/pubmed/16497993

[5] Sampson UKA, Norman PE, Fowkes FGR, Aboyans V, Song Y, Harrell FE, et al. Global and regional burden of aortic dissection and aneurysms: Mortality trends in 21 world regions, 1990 to 2010. Vol. 9, *Global Heart*. Elsevier B.V.; 2014. p. 171-180.e10.

[6] Kuivaniemi H, Platsoucas chris d, Tilson MD. *Aortic Aneurysms: an Immune Disease with a Strong Genetic Component*. Circulation [Internet]. 2008 Jan 15;117(2):242–52. Available from: http://www.ncbi.nlm.nih.gov/pubmed/18195185

[7] Harky A, Fan KS, Kwok HT, Chan J. Local Anaesthetic Technique in Endovascular Abdominal Aortic Aneurysm Repair: Is it Time to Change the Paradigm? *J Vasc Med Surg*. 2018;06(06).

[8] Harky A, Fok M, Fraser H, Howard C, Rimmer L, Bashir M. Could cerebrospinal fluid biomarkers offer better predictive value for spinal

cord ischaemia than current neuromonitoring techniques during thoracoabdominal aortic aneurysm repair – a systematic review. *Brazilian J Cardiovasc Surg.* 2019;34(4):464–71.

[9] Collins JA, Munoz JV, Patel TR, Loukas M, Tubbs RS. The anatomy of the aging aorta. Vol. 27, *Clinical Anatomy*. Wiley-Liss Inc.; 2014. p. 463–6.

[10] Harky A, Fan KS, Fan KH. The genetics and biomechanics of thoracic aortic diseases. *Vasc Biol.* 2019 Oct 16;

[11] Agaimy A, Weyand M, Strecker T. Inflammatory thoracic aortic aneurysm (lymphoplasmacytic thoracic aortitis): a 13-year-experience at a German Heart Center with emphasis on possible role of IgG4. *Int J Clin Exp Pathol* [Internet]. 2013;6(9):1713–22. Available from: http://www.ncbi.nlm.nih.gov/pubmed/24040436

[12] Kuivaniemi H, Ryer EJ, Elmore JR, Tromp G. Understanding the pathogenesis of abdominal aortic aneurysms. Vol. 13, *Expert Review of Cardiovascular Therapy*. Taylor and Francis Ltd; 2015. p. 975–87.

[13] Quintana RA, Taylor WR. Cellular Mechanisms of Aortic Aneurysm Formation. *Circ Res.* 2019 Feb 15;124(4):607–18.

[14] Xiao TS. Innate immunity and inflammation. Vol. 14, Cellular and Molecular Immunology. *Chinese Soc Immunology*; 2017. p. 1–3.

[15] Yan H, Cui B, Zhang X, Fu X, Yan J, Wang X, et al. Antagonism of toll-like receptor 2 attenuates the formation and progression of abdominal aortic aneurysm. *Acta Pharm Sin B.* 2015 May 1;5(3):176–87.

[16] Harja E, Bu DX, Hudson BI, Jong SC, Shen X, Hallam K, et al. Vascular and inflammatory stresses mediate atherosclerosis via RAGE and its ligands in apoE-/- mice. *J Clin Invest.* 2008 Jan 2;118(1):183–94.

[17] Lotze MT, Zeh HJ, Rubartelli A, Sparvero LJ, Amoscato AA, Washburn NR, et al. The grateful dead: Damage-associated molecular pattern molecules and reduction/oxidation regulate immunity. Vol. 220, *Immunological Reviews*. 2007. p. 60–81.

[18] Hou B, Reizis B, DeFranco AL. Toll-like Receptors Activate Innate and Adaptive Immunity by using Dendritic Cell-Intrinsic and -Extrinsic Mechanisms. *Immunity*. 2008 Aug 15;29(2):272–82.

[19] Furusho A, Aoki H, Ohno-Urabe S, Nishihara M, Hirakata S, Nishida N, et al. Involvement of B cells, immunoglobulins, and syk in the pathogenesis of abdominal aortic aneurysm. *J Am Heart Assoc*. 2018 Mar 20;7(6).

[20] Zhang L, Wang Y. B lymphocytes in abdominal aortic aneurysms. Vol. 242, *Atherosclerosis*. Elsevier Ireland Ltd; 2015. p. 311–7.

[21] Raffort J, Lareyre F, Clément M, Hassen-Khodja R, Chinetti G, Mallat Z. Monocytes and macrophages in abdominal aortic aneurysm. Vol. 14, *Nature Reviews Cardiology*. Nature Publishing Group; 2017. p. 457–71.

[22] Pyo R, Lee JK, Shipley JM, Curci JA, Mao D, Ziporin SJ, et al. Targeted gene disruption of matrix metalloproteinase-9 (gelatinase B) suppresses development of experimental abdominal aortic aneurysms. *J Clin Invest*. 2000;105(11):1641–9.

[23] Longo GM, Xiong W, Greiner TC, Zhao Y, Fiotti N, Baxter BT. Matrix metalloproteinases 2 and 9 work in concert to produce aortic aneurysms. *J Clin Invest* [Internet]. 2002 Sep 1;110(5):625–32. Available from: http://www.jci.org/articles/view/15334

[24] Longo GM, Buda SJ, Fiotta N, Xiong W, Griener T, Shapiro S, et al. MMP-12 has a role in abdominal aortic aneurysms in mice. *Surgery*. 2005;137(4):457–62.

[25] Qin Y, Cao X, Guo J, Zhang Y, Pan L, Zhang H, et al. Deficiency of cathepsin S attenuates angiotensin II-induced abdominal aortic aneurysm formation in apolipoprotein E-deficient mice. *Cardiovasc Res*. 2012 Dec 1;96(3):401–10.

[26] Eskandari MK, Vijungco JD, Flores A, Borensztajn J, Shively V, Pearce WH. Enhanced abdominal aortic aneurysm in TIMP-1-deficient mice. *J Surg Res*. 2005 Feb;123(2):289–93.

[27] Dale MA, Ruhlman MK, Baxter BT. Inflammatory cell phenotypes in AAAs: Their role and potential as targets for therapy. *Arterioscler Thromb Vasc Biol*. 2015 Aug 25;35(8):1746–55.

[28] Amento EP, Ehsani N, Palmer H, Libby P. Cytokines and growth factors positively and negatively regulate interstitial collagen gene expression in human vascular smooth muscle cells. *Arterioscler Thromb a J Vasc Biol* [Internet]. 11(5):1223–30. Available from: http://www.ncbi.nlm.nih.gov/pubmed/1911708

[29] Atri C, Guerfali FZ, Laouini D. Role of human macrophage polarization in inflammation during infectious diseases. Vol. 19, *International Journal of Molecular Sciences*. MDPI AG; 2018.

[30] Andreata F, Syvannarath V, Clement M, Delbosc S, Guedj K, Fornasa G, et al. Macrophage CD31 Signaling in Dissecting Aortic Aneurysm. *J Am Coll Cardiol*. 2018 Jul 3;72(1):45–57.

[31] Kong DH, Kim YK, Kim MR, Jang JH, Lee S. Emerging roles of vascular cell adhesion molecule-1 (VCAM-1) in immunological disorders and cancer. Vol. 19, *International Journal of Molecular Sciences*. MDPI AG; 2018.

[32] Boytard L, Spear R, Chinetti-Gbaguidi G, Acosta-Martin AE, Vanhoutte J, Lamblin N, et al. Role of proinflammatory CD68+ mannose receptor-macrophages in peroxiredoxin-1 expression and in abdominal aortic aneurysms in humans. *Arterioscler Thromb Vasc Biol*. 2013 Feb;33(2):431–8.

[33] Beyer M, Mallmann MR, Xue J, Staratschek-Jox A, Vorholt D, Krebs W, et al. High-Resolution Transcriptome of Human Macrophages. *PLoS One*. 2012 Sep 21;7(9).

[34] Vogel DYS, Glim JE, Stavenuiter AWD, Breur M, Heijnen P, Amor S, et al. Human macrophage polarization in vitro: Maturation and activation methods compared. *Immunobiology*. 2014;219(9):695–703.

[35] Italiani P, Mazza EMC, Lucchesi D, Cifola I, Gemelli C, Grande A, et al. Transcriptomic Profiling of the Development of the Inflammatory Response in Human Monocytes In Vitro. Poli G, editor. *PLoS One* [Internet]. 2014 Feb 3;9(2):e87680. Available from: https://dx.plos.org/10.1371/journal.pone.0087680

[36] Martinez FO, Gordon S, Locati M, Mantovani A. Transcriptional Profiling of the Human Monocyte-to-Macrophage Differentiation and

Polarization: New Molecules and Patterns of Gene Expression. *J Immunol.* 2006 Nov 15;177(10):7303–11.

[37] Cheng Z, Zhou YZ, Wu Y, Wu QY, Liao XB, Fu XM, et al. Diverse roles of macrophage polarization in aortic aneurysm: destruction and repair [Internet]. *Journal of Translational Medicine BioMed Central Ltd.*; Dec 13, 2018 p. 354. Available from: https://translational-medicine.biomedcentral.com/articles/10.1186/s12967-018-1731-0

[38] Moore JP, Vinh A, Tuck KL, Sakkal S, Krishnan SM, Chan CT, et al. M2 macrophage accumulation in the aortic wall during angiotensin ii infusion in mice is associated with fibrosis, elastin loss, and elevated blood pressure. *Am J Physiol - Hear Circ Physiol.* 2015 Sep 3;309(5):H906–17.

[39] Hans CP, Koenig SN, Huang N, Cheng J, Beceiro S, Guggilam A, et al. Inhibition of Notch1 signaling reduces abdominal aortic aneurysm in mice by attenuating macrophage-mediated inflammation. *Arterioscler Thromb Vasc Biol.* 2012 Dec;32(12):3012–23.

[40] Xu H, Zhu J, Smith S, Foldi J, Zhao B, Chung AY, et al. Notch-RBP-J signaling regulates the transcription factor IRF8 to promote inflammatory macrophage polarization. *Nat Immunol.* 2012 Jul;13(7):642–50.

[41] McCormick ML, Gavrila D, Weintraub NL. Role of oxidative stress in the pathogenesis of abdominal aortic aneurysms. Vol. 27, *Arteriosclerosis, Thrombosis, and Vascular Biology.* 2007. p. 461–9.

[42] Ley K, Miller YI, Hedrick CC. Monocyte and macrophage dynamics during atherogenesis. Vol. 31, *Arteriosclerosis, Thrombosis, and Vascular Biology.* 2011. p. 1506–16.

[43] Petersen E, Wågberg F, Ängquist KA. Serum concentrations of elastin-derived peptides in patients with specific manifestations of atherosclerotic disease. *Eur J Vasc Endovasc Surg.* 2002;24(5):440–4.

[44] Dale MA, Xiong W, Carson JS, Suh MK, Karpisek AD, Meisinger TM, et al. Elastin-Derived Peptides Promote Abdominal Aortic Aneurysm Formation by Modulating M1/M2 Macrophage Polarization. *J Immunol.* 2016 Jun 1;196(11):4536–43.

[45] Ishibashi M, Egashira K, Zhao Q, Hiasa K ichi, Ohtani K, Ihara Y, et al. Bone marrow-derived monocyte chemoattractant protein-1 receptor CCR2 is critical in angiotensin II-induced acceleration of atherosclerosis and aneurysm formation in hypercholesterolemic mice. *Arterioscler Thromb Vasc Biol.* 2004;24(11).

[46] Tsou CL, Peters W, Si Y, Slaymaker S, Aslanian AM, Weisberg SP, et al. Critical roles for CCR2 and MCP-3 in monocyte mobilization from bone marrow and recruitment to inflammatory sites. *J Clin Invest.* 2007 Apr 2;117(4):902–9.

[47] Moran CS, Jose RJ, Moxon J V., Roomberg A, Norman PE, Rush C, et al. Everolimus limits aortic aneurysm in the apolipoprotein e-deficient mouse by downregulating C-C chemokine receptor 2 positive monocytes. *Arterioscler Thromb Vasc Biol.* 2013 Apr;33(4):814–21.

[48] Baohui Xu, Naoki Fujimura, Haojun Xuan, Jackson Dalman, Yuko Furisho, Hiroki Tanaka, Keith Glover, Martin Rouer, Kohji Aoyama, Sara Michie and RD. Chemokine Receptor CCR2 Mediates Monocyte Mobilization and Migration in Experimental Aneurysms. *Arterioscler Thromb Vasc Biol.* 2018;

[49] de Waard V, Bot I, de Jager SCA, Talib S, Egashira K, de Vries MR, et al. Systemic MCP1/CCR2 blockade and leukocyte specific MCP1/CCR2 inhibition affect aortic aneurysm formation differently. *Atherosclerosis.* 2010 Jul;211(1):84–9.

[50] Uchida W, Narita Y, Yamawaki-Ogata A, Tokuda Y, Mutsuga M, Lee Fujimoto K, et al. The oral administration of clarithromycin prevents the progression and rupture of aortic aneurysm. *J Vasc Surg.* 2018 Dec 1;68(6):82S-92S.e2.

[51] Calder PC. Polyunsaturated fatty acids, inflammation, and immunity. *Lipids.* 2001;36(9):1007–24.

[52] Yoshihara T, Shimada K, Fukao K, Sai E, Sato-Okabayashi Y, Matsumori R, et al. Omega 3 polyunsaturated fatty acids suppress the development of aortic aneurysms through the inhibition of macrophage-mediated inflammation. *Circ J.* 2015 Jun 9;79(7):1470–8.

[53] Mantovani A, Cassatella MA, Costantini C, Jaillon S. Neutrophils in the activation and regulation of innate and adaptive immunity. Vol. 11, *Nature Reviews Immunology*. 2011. p. 519–31.

[54] Selders GS, Fetz AE, Radic MZ, Bowlin GL. An overview of the role of neutrophils in innate immunity, inflammation and host-biomaterial integration. *Regen Biomater*. 2017;4(1):55–68.

[55] Perobelli SM, Galvani RG, Gonçalves-Silva T, Xavier CR, Nóbrega A, Bonomo A. Plasticity of neutrophils reveals modulatory capacity. *Brazilian J Med Biol Res*. 2015 Aug 1;48(8):665–75.

[56] Björnsdottir H, Welin A, Michaëlsson E, Osla V, Berg S, Christenson K, et al. Neutrophil NET formation is regulated from the inside by myeloperoxidase-processed reactive oxygen species. *Free Radic Biol Med*. 2015 Dec 1;89:1024–35.

[57] Lópcz-Boado YS, Espinola M, Bahr S, Belaaouaj A. Neutrophil Serine Proteinases Cleave Bacterial Flagellin, Abrogating Its Host Response-Inducing Activity. *J Immunol*. 2004 Jan 1;172(1):509–15.

[58] Meher AK, Spinosa M, Davis JP, Pope N, Laubach VE, Su G, et al. Novel Role of IL (Interleukin)-1β in Neutrophil Extracellular Trap Formation and Abdominal Aortic Aneurysms. *Arterioscler Thromb Vasc Biol* [Internet]. 2018;38(4):843–53. Available from: http://www.ncbi.nlm.nih.gov/pubmed/29472233

[59] Li H, Bai S, Ao Q, Wang X, Tian X, Li X, et al. Modulation of immune-inflammatory responses in abdominal aortic aneurysm: Emerging molecular targets. Vol. 2018, *Journal of Immunology Research*. Hindawi Limited; 2018.

[60] Eliason JL, Hannawa KK, Ailawadi G, Sinha I, Ford JW, Deogracias MP, et al. *Neutrophil depletion inhibits experimental abdominal aortic aneurysm formation*. Circulation [Internet]. 2005 Jul 12;112(2):232–40. Available from: http://www.ncbi.nlm.nih.gov/pubmed/16009808

[61] Houard X, Touat Z, Ollivier V, Louedec L, Philippe M, Sebbag U, et al. Mediators of neutrophil recruitment in human abdominal aortic aneurysms. *Cardiovasc Res*. 2009 Jun;82(3):532–41.

[62] Ramos-Mozo P, Madrigal-Matute J, Vega de Ceniga M, Blanco-Colio LM, Meilhac O, Feldman L, et al. Increased plasma levels of NGAL, a marker of neutrophil activation, in patients with abdominal aortic aneurysm. *Atherosclerosis*. 2012 Feb;220(2):552–6.

[63] Adkison AM, Raptis SZ, Kelley DG, Pham CTN. Dipeptidyl peptidase I activates neutrophil-derived serine proteases and regulates the development of acute experimental arthritis. *J Clin Invest* [Internet]. 2002 Feb 1;109(3):363–71. Available from: http://www.jci.org/articles/view/13462

[64] Pagano MB, Bartoli MA, Ennis TL, Mao D, Simmons PM, Thompson RW, et al. Critical role of dipeptidyl peptidase I in neutrophil recruitment during the development of experimental abdominal aortic aneurysms. *Proc Natl Acad Sci U S A*. 2007 Feb 20;104(8):2855–60.

[65] Pham CTN. Neutrophil serine proteases: Specific regulators of inflammation. Vol. 6, *Nature Reviews Immunology*. 2006. p. 541–50.

[66] Fadok VA, Bratton DL, Guthrie L, Henson PM. Differential Effects of Apoptotic Versus Lysed Cells on Macrophage Production of Cytokines: Role of Proteases. *J Immunol*. 2001 Jun 1;166(11):6847–54.

[67] Yan H, Zhou HF, Akk A, Hu Y, Springer LE, Ennis TL, et al. Neutrophil Proteases Promote Experimental Abdominal Aortic Aneurysm via Extracellular Trap Release and Plasmacytoid Dendritic Cell Activation. *Arterioscler Thromb Vasc Biol*. 2016 Aug 1;36(8):1660–9.

[68] Wilson WRW, Schwalbe EC, Jones JL, Bell PRF, Thompson MM. Matrix metalloproteinase 8 (neutrophil collagenase) in the pathogenesis of abdominal aortic aneurysm. *Br J Surg* [Internet]. 2005 Jul;92(7):828–33. Available from: http://doi.wiley.com/10.1002/bjs.4993

[69] Kurihara T, Shimizu-Hirota R, Shimoda M, Adachi T, Shimizu H, Weiss SJ, et al. *Neutrophil-derived matrix metalloproteinase 9 triggers acute aortic dissection*. Circulation [Internet]. 2012 Dec 18;126(25):3070–80. Available from: http://www.ncbi.nlm.nih.gov/pubmed/23136157

[70] Anzai A, Shimoda M, Endo J, Kohno T, Katsumata Y, Matsuhashi T, et al. Adventitial CXCL1/G-CSF expression in response to acute aortic dissection triggers local neutrophil recruitment and activation leading to aortic rupture. *Circ Res* [Internet]. 2015 Feb 13;116(4):612–23. Available from: http://www.ncbi.nlm.nih.gov/pubmed/25563839

[71] Fontaine V, Jacob MP, Houard X, Rossignol P, Plissonnier D, Angles-Cano E, et al. Involvement of the mural thrombus as a site of protease release and activation in human aortic aneurysms. *Am J Pathol.* 2002;161(5):1701–10.

[72] Hance KA, Tataria M, Ziporin SJ, Lee JK, Thompson RW. Monocyte chemotactic activity in human abdominal aortic aneurysms: Role of elastin degradation peptides and the 67-kD cell surface elastin receptor. *J Vasc Surg.* 2002;35(2):254–61.

[73] Senior RM, Griffin GL, Mecham RP, Wrenn DS, Prasad KU, Urry DW. Val-Gly-Val-Ala-Pro-Gly, a repeating peptide in elastin, is chemotactic for fibroblasts and monocytes. *J Cell Biol.* 1984;99(3):870–4.

[74] Nowak D, Głowczyńska I, Piasecka G. Chemotactic activity of elastin-derived peptides for human polymorphonuclear leukocytes and their effect on hydrogen peroxide and myeloperoxidase release. *Arch Immunol Ther Exp (Warsz)* [Internet]. 1989;37(5–6):741–8. Available from: http://www.ncbi.nlm.nih.gov/pubmed/2562130

[75] Kim HW, Blomkalns AL, Ogbi M, Thomas M, Gavrila D, Neltner BS, et al. Role of myeloperoxidase in abdominal aortic aneurysm formation: Mitigation by taurine. *Am J Physiol - Hear Circ Physiol.* 2017 Dec 1;313(6):H1168–79.

[76] Stone KD, Prussin C, Metcalfe DD. IgE, mast cells, basophils, and eosinophils. *J Allergy Clin Immunol.* 2010 Feb;125(2 SUPPL. 2).

[77] Tsuruda T, Kato J, Hatakeyama K, Kojima K, Yano M, Yano Y, et al. Adventitial mast cells contribute to pathogenesis in the progression of abdominal aortic aneurysm. *Circ Res* [Internet]. 2008 Jun 6;102(11):1368–77. Available from: http://www.ncbi.nlm.nih.gov/pubmed/18451339

[78] Sun J, Sukhova GK, Yang M, Wolters PJ, MacFarlane LA, Libby P, et al. Mast cells modulate the pathogenesis of elastase-induced abdominal aortic aneurysms in mice. *J Clin Invest.* 2007 Nov 1;117(11):3359–68.

[79] Gozalo AS, Elkins WR, Lambert LE. Eosinophilic aortitis with thoracic aortic aneurysm and rupture in a captive-born owl monkey. *J Med Primatol.* 2018 Dec 1;47(6):423–6.

[80] Shah AD, Denaxas S, Nicholas O, Hingorani AD, Hemingway H. Low eosinophil and low lymphocyte counts and the incidence of 12 cardiovascular diseases: A CALIBER cohort study. *Open Hear.* 2016 Sep 1;3(2).

[81] Liu C-L, Wemmelund H, Wang Y, Liao M, Lindholt JS, Johnsen SP, et al. Asthma Associates With Human Abdominal Aortic Aneurysm and Rupture. *Arterioscler Thromb Vasc Biol* [Internet]. 2016 Mar;36(3):570–8. Available from: http://www.ncbi.nlm.nih.gov/pubmed/26868210

[82] Mellman I. Dendritic cells: master regulators of the immune response. Vol. 1, *Cancer immunology research.* 2013. p. 145–9.

[83] Bobryshev Y V., Lord RSA. Ultrastructural Recognition of Cells with Dendritic Cell Morphology in Human Aortic Intima. Contacting Interactions of Vascular Dendritic Cells in Athero-resistant and Athero-prone Areas of the Normal Aorta. *Arch Histol Cytol.* 1995;58(3):307–22.

[84] Bobryshev Y V., Lord RSA. Langhans cells of human arterial intima: Uniform by stellate appearance but different by nature. *Tissue Cell.* 1996;28(2):177–94.

[85] Zhao L, Moos MPW, Gräbner R, Pédrono F, Fan J, Kaiser B, et al. The 5-lipoxygenase pathway promotes pathogenesis of hyperlipidemia- dependent aortic aneurysm. *Nat Med.* 2004 Sep;10(9):966–73.

[86] Ludewig B, Freigang S, Jäggi M, Kurrer MO, Pei YC, Vlk L, et al. Linking immune-mediated arterial inflammation and cholesterol-induced atherosclerosis in a transgenic mouse model. *Proc Natl Acad Sci U S A.* 2000 Nov 7;97(23):12752–7.

[87] Manthey HD, Zernecke A. Dendritic cells in atherosclerosis: Functions in immune regulation and beyond. *Thromb Haemost.* 2011 Nov;106(5):772–8.

[88] Niessner A, Sato K, Chaikof EL, Colmegna I, Goronzy JJ, Weyand CM. Pathogen-sensing plasmacytoid dendritic cells stimulate cytotoxic T-cell function in the atherosclerotic plaque through interferon-α. *Circulation.* 2006 Dec;114(23):2482–9.

[89] Lewis JS, Dolgova N V., Chancellor TJ, Acharya AP, Karpiak J V., Lele TP, et al. The effect of cyclic mechanical strain on activation of dendritic cells cultured on adhesive substrates. *Biomaterials.* 2013 Dec;34(36):9063–70.

[90] Dennison AR, Watkins RM, Gunning AJ. Simultaneous aortic and pulmonary artery aneurysms due to giant cell arteritis. *Thorax* [Internet]. 1985;40(2):156–7. Available from: http://thorax.bmj.com/

[91] Sagan A, Mikolajczyk TP, Mrowiecki W, MacRitchie N, Daly K, Meldrum A, et al. T Cells Are Dominant Population in Human Abdominal Aortic Aneurysms and Their Infiltration in the Perivascular Tissue Correlates With Disease Severity. *Front Immunol* [Internet]. 2019 Sep 4;10. Available from: https://www.frontiersin.org/article/10.3389/fimmu.2019.01979/full

[92] Amin HZ, Sasaki N, Yamashita T, Mizoguchi T, Hayashi T, Emoto T, et al. CTLA-4 Protects against Angiotensin II-Induced Abdominal Aortic Aneurysm Formation in Mice. *Sci Rep.* 2019 Dec 1;9(1).

[93] NK, γδ T and NKT Cells. In: *Primer to the Immune Response.* Elsevier; 2014. p. 247–68.

[94] Xiong W, Zhao Y, Prall A, Greiner TC, Baxter BT. Key Roles of CD4 + T Cells and IFN-γ in the Development of Abdominal Aortic Aneurysms in a Murine Model. *J Immunol.* 2004 Feb 15;172(4):2607–12.

[95] Kasashima S, Kawashima A, Zen Y, Ozaki S, Kasashima F, Endo M, et al. Upregulated interleukins (IL-6, IL-10, and IL-13) in immunoglobulin G4-related aortic aneurysm patients. *J Vasc Surg.* 2018 Apr 1;67(4):1248–62.

[96] King VL, Lin AY, Kristo F, Anderson TJT, Ahluwalia N, Hardy GJ, et al. Interferon-γ and the interferon-inducible chemokine CXCL10 protect against aneurysm formation and rupture. *Circulation*. 2009 Jan 27;119(3):426–35.

[97] Shimizu K, Shichiri M, Libby P, Lee R, Mitchell R. Th2-predominant inflammation and blockade of IFN-γ signaling induce aneurysms in allografted aortas. *J Clin Invest*. 2004;114(2):300–8.

[98] Ye J, Wang Y, Wang Z, Ji Q, Huang Y, Zeng T, et al. Circulating Th1, Th2, Th9, Th17, Th22, and Treg levels in aortic dissection patients. *Mediators Inflamm*. 2018;2018.

[99] Wei Z, Wang Y, Zhang K, Liao Y, Ye P, Wu J, et al. Inhibiting the Th17/IL-17A-related inflammatory responses with digoxin confers protection against experimental abdominal aortic aneurysm. *Arterioscler Thromb Vasc Biol* [Internet]. 2014 Nov;34(11):2429–38. Available from: http://www.ncbi.nlm.nih.gov/pubmed/25234817

[100] Kyaw T, Winship A, Tay C, Kanellakis P, Hosseini H, Cao A, et al. Cytotoxic and proinflammatory CD8+ T lymphocytes promote development of vulnerable atherosclerotic plaques in ApoE-deficient mice. *Circulation*. 2013 Mar 5;127(9):1028–39.

[101] Zhou H, Yan H, Cannon JL, Springer LE, Green JM, Pham CTN. CD43-Mediated IFN-γ Production by CD8 + T Cells Promotes Abdominal Aortic Aneurysm in Mice. *J Immunol*. 2013 May 15;190(10):5078–85.

[102] Gijs H van Puijvelde, Amanda C Foks, Ilze Bot, Kim L Habets, Saskia C de Jager, Mariette N ter Borg, Theo J van Berkel, Paul Quax and JK. Abstract 153: NKT Cells Aggravate the Development of Abdominal Aortic Aneurysms. *Arterioscler Thromb Vasc Biol*. 2018;

[103] van Puijvelde GHM, Kuiper J. NKT cells in cardiovascular diseases. *Eur J Pharmacol*. 2017 Dec 5;816:47–57.

[104] Chan WL, Pejnovic N, Hamilton H, Liew TV, Popadic D, Poggi A, et al. Atherosclerotic abdominal aortic aneurysm and the interaction between autologous human plaque-derived vascular smooth muscle cells, type 1 NKT, and helper T cells. *Circ Res* [Internet]. 2005 Apr

1;96(6):675–83. Available from: http://www.ncbi.nlm.nih.gov/pubmed/15731463

[105] Chan WL, Pejnovic N, Liew TV, Hamilton H. Predominance of Th2 response in human abdominal aortic aneurysm: Mistaken identity for IL-4-producing NK and NKT cells? In: *Cellular Immunology*. 2005. p. 109–14.

[106] Lu S, White J V., Lin WL, Zhang X, Solomides C, Evans K, et al. Aneurysmal Lesions of Patients with Abdominal Aortic Aneurysm Contain Clonally Expanded T Cells. *J Immunol*. 2014 May 15;192(10):4897–912.

[107] Platsoucas CD, Lu S, Nwaneshiudu I, Solomides C, Agelan A, Ntaoula N, et al. Abdominal aortic aneurysm is a specific antigen-driven T cell disease. In: *Annals of the New York Academy of Sciences*. Blackwell Publishing Inc.; 2006. p. 224–35.

[108] Zhang S, Kan X, Li Y, Li P, Zhang C, Li G, et al. Deficiency of γδT cells protects against abdominal aortic aneurysms by regulating phosphoinositide 3-kinase/AKT signaling. *J Vasc Surg*. 2018 Mar 1;67(3):899-908.e1.

[109] Galle C, Schandené L, Stordeur P, Peignois Y, Ferreira J, Wautrecht JC, et al. Predominance of type 1 CD4+ T cells in human abdominal aortic aneurysm. *Clin Exp Immunol*. 2005 Dec;142(3):519–27.

[110] Téo FH, De Oliveira RTD, Villarejos L, Mamoni RL, Altemani A, Menezes FH, et al. Characterization of CD4 + T cell subsets in patients with abdominal aortic aneurysms. *Mediators Inflamm*. 2018;2018.

[111] Galle C, Schandené L, Ferreira J, Wautrecht JC, Dereume JP, Goldman M. T-cell phenotype and polarization in human abdominal aortic aneurysm. *J Mal Vasc*. 2004;

[112] Ait-Oufella H, Wang Y, Herbin O, Bourcier S, Potteaux S, Joffre J, et al. Natural regulatory T cells limit angiotensin II-induced aneurysm formation and rupture in mice. *Arterioscler Thromb Vasc Biol*. 2013 Oct;33(10):2374–9.

[113] Ohkura N, Kitagawa Y, Sakaguchi S. Development and Maintenance of Regulatory T cells. Vol. 38, *Immunity*. 2013. p. 414–23.

[114] Wang Y, Ait-Oufella H, Herbin O, Bonnin P, Ramkhelawon B, Taleb S, et al. *TGF-beta Activity Protects Against Inflammatory Aortic Aneurysm Progression and Complications in Angiotensin II-infused Mice.* 2010 Feb 1;120(2). Available from: http://www.ncbi.nlm.nih.gov/pubmed/20101093

[115] Gao F, Chambon P, Offermanns S, Tellides G, Kong W, Zhang X, et al. Disruption of TGF-β signaling in smooth muscle cell prevents elastase-induced abdominal aortic aneurysm. *Biochem Biophys Res Commun.* 2014 Nov 7;454(1):137–43.

[116] Hoffman W, Lakkis FG, Chalasani G. B cells, antibodies, and more. *Clin J Am Soc Nephrol.* 2016 Jan 7;11(1):137–54.

[117] Grönwall C, Vas J, Silverman GJ. Protective roles of natural IgM antibodies. Vol. 3, *Frontiers in Immunology*. 2012.

[118] Bobryshev Y V., Lord RSA. Vascular-associated lymphoid tissue (VALT) involvement in aortic aneurysm. *Atherosclerosis*. 2001;154(1):15–21.

[119] Meher AK, Johnston WF, Lu G, Pope NH, Bhamidipati CM, Harmon DB, et al. B2 cells suppress experimental abdominal aortic aneurysms. *Am J Pathol.* 2014 Nov 1;184(11):3130–41.

[120] Schaheen B, Downs EA, Serbulea V, Almenara CCP, Spinosa M, Su G, et al. B-Cell Depletion Promotes Aortic Infiltration of Immunosuppressive Cells and Is Protective of Experimental Aortic Aneurysm. *Arterioscler Thromb Vasc Biol* [Internet]. 2016;36(11):2191–202. Available from: http://www.ncbi.nlm.nih.gov/pubmed/27634836

[121] DiLillo DJ, Hamaguchi Y, Ueda Y, Yang K, Uchida J, Haas KM, et al. Maintenance of Long-Lived Plasma Cells and Serological Memory Despite Mature and Memory B Cell Depletion during CD20 Immunotherapy in Mice. *J Immunol.* 2008 Jan 1;180(1):361–71.

[122] Kasashima S, Zen Y. IgG4-related inflammatory abdominal aortic aneurysm. *Curr Opin Rheumatol* [Internet]. 2011 Jan;23(1):18–23. Available from: https://insights.ovid.com/crossref?an=00002281-201101000-00005

[123] Perugino CA, Wallace ZS, Meyersohn N, Oliveira G, Stone JR, Stone JH. Large vessel involvement by IgG4-related disease. *Med* (United States). 2016 Jul 1;95(28).

[124] Hourai R, Kasashima S, Sohmiya K, Yamauchi Y, Ozawa H, Hirose Y, et al. IgG4-positive cell infiltration in various cardiovascular disorders - results from histopathological analysis of surgical samples. *BMC Cardiovasc Disord* [Internet]. 2017 Dec 3;17(1):52. Available from: http://bmccardiovascdisord.biomedcentral.com/articles/10.1186/s12872-017-0488-3

[125] Tuleta I, Skowasch D, Aurich F, Eckstein N, Schueler R, Pizarro C, et al. Asthma is associated with atherosclerotic artery changes. Feng Y-M, editor. *PLoS One* [Internet]. 2017 Oct 26;12(10):e0186820. Available from: http://dx.plos.org/10.1371/journal.pone.0186820

[126] Abd-Elmoniem KZ, Ramos N, Yazdani SK, Ghanem AM, Holland SM, Freeman AF, et al. Coronary atherosclerosis and dilation in hyper IgE syndrome patients: Depiction by magnetic resonance vessel wall imaging and pathological correlation. *Atherosclerosis*. 2017 Mar 1;258:20–5.

[127] Tsiantoulas D, Bot I, Ozsvar-Kozma M, Göderle L, Perkmann T, Hartvigsen K, et al. Increased Plasma IgE Accelerate Atherosclerosis in Secreted IgM Deficiency. *Circ Res* [Internet]. 2017 Jan 6;120(1):78–84. Available from: http://www.ncbi.nlm.nih.gov/pubmed/27903567

[128] Freeman AF, Avila EM, Shaw PA, Davis J, Hsu AP, Welch P, et al. Coronary artery abnormalities in hyper-IgE syndrome. *J Clin Immunol*. 2011 Jun;31(3):338–45.

[129] Wang J, Lindholt JS, Sukhova GK, Shi MA, Xia M, Chen H, et al. IgE actions on <scp>CD</scp> 4 + T cells, mast cells, and macrophages participate in the pathogenesis of experimental abdominal aortic aneurysms. *EMBO Mol Med* [Internet]. 2014 Jul 24;6(7):952–69. Available from: https://onlinelibrary.wiley.com/doi/abs/10.15252/emmm.201303811

[130] Pasquinelli G, Preda P, Gargiulo M, Vici M, Cenacchi G, Stella A, et al. An immunohistochemical study of inflammatory abdominal aortic aneurysms. *J Submicrosc Cytol Pathol*. 1993;25(1):103–12.

[131] Villar LM, Casanova B, Ouamara N, Comabella M, Jalili F, Leppert D, et al. Immunoglobulin M oligoclonal bands: Biomarker of targetable inflammation in primary progressive multiple sclerosis. *Ann Neurol* [Internet]. 2014 Aug;76(2):231–40. Available from: http://doi.wiley.com/10.1002/ana.24190

[132] Gleissner CA, Erbel C, Haeussler J, Akhavanpoor M, Domschke G, Linden F, et al. Low levels of natural IgM antibodies against phosphorylcholine are independently associated with vascular remodeling in patients with coronary artery disease. *Clin Res Cardiol*. 2014;104(1):13–22.

[133] Kyaw T, Tipping P, Bobik A, Toh BH. Protective Role of Natural IgM-Producing B1a Cells in Atherosclerosis. Vol. 22, *Trends in Cardiovascular Medicine*. 2012. p. 48–53.

[134] Spits H, Cupedo T. Innate Lymphoid Cells: Emerging Insights in Development, Lineage Relationships, and Function. *Annu Rev Immunol*. 2012 Apr 23;30(1):647–75.

[135] Nau D, Altmayer N, Mattner J. Mechanisms of innate lymphoid cell and natural killer t cell activation during mucosal inflammation. Vol. 2014, *Journal of Immunology Research*. Hindawi Publishing Corporation; 2014.

[136] Cella M, Gamini R, Sécca C, Collins PL, Zhao S, Peng V, et al. Subsets of ILC3−ILC1-like cells generate a diversity spectrum of innate lymphoid cells in human mucosal tissues. *Nat Immunol*. 2019 Aug 1;20(8):980–91.

[137] Seko Y, Sato O, Takagi A, Tada Y, Matsuo H, Yagita H, et al. Perforin-Secreting Killer Cell Infiltration in the Aortic Tissue of Patients With Atherosclerotic Aortic Aneurysm. *Jpn Circ J* [Internet]. 1997;61(12):965–70. Available from: http://joi.jlc.jst.go.jp/JST.JSTAGE/jcj/61.965?from=CrossRef

[138] Forester ND, Cruickshank SM, Scott DJA, Carding SR. Increased natural killer cell activity in patients with an abdominal aortic aneurysm. *Br J Surg.* 2006 Jan;93(1):46–54.

[139] Martínez-Rodríguez JE, Munné-Collado J, Rasal R, Cuadrado E, Roig L, Ois A, et al. Expansion of the NKG2C+ natural killer-cell subset is associated with high-risk carotid atherosclerotic plaques in seropositive patients for human cytomegalovirus. *Arterioscler Thromb Vasc Biol.* 2013 Nov;33(11):2653–9.

[140] Selathurai A, Deswaerte V, Kanellakis P, Tipping P, Toh BH, Bobik A, et al. Natural killer (NK) cells augment atherosclerosis by cytotoxic-dependent mechanisms. *Cardiovasc Res.* 2014;102(1):128–37.

[141] Li J, Xia N, Wen S, Li D, Lu Y, Gu M, et al. IL (Interleukin)-33 Suppresses Abdominal Aortic Aneurysm by Enhancing Regulatory T-Cell Expansion and Activity. *Arterioscler Thromb Vasc Biol.* 2019 Mar 1;39(3):446–58.

[142] Molofsky AB, Van Gool F, Liang HE, Van Dyken SJ, Nussbaum JC, Lee J, et al. InterleuKin-33 And Interferon-Γ Counter-Regulate Group 2 Innate Lymphoid Cell Activation During Immune Perturbation. *Immunity.* 2015 Jul 21;43(1):161–74.

[143] Newland SA, Mohanta S, Clément M, Taleb S, Walker JA, Nus M, et al. Type-2 innate lymphoid cells control the development of atherosclerosis in mice. *Nat Commun.* 2017 Jun 7;8.

[144] *TLR2 toll like receptor 2 [Homo sapiens (human)] - Gene - NCBI* [Internet]. Available from: https://www.ncbi.nlm.nih.gov/gene/7097

[145] Oliveira-Nascimento L, Massari P, Wetzler LM. The role of TLR2 ininfection and immunity. Vol. 3, *Frontiers in Immunology.* 2012.

[146] Franchi L, Warner N, Viani K, Nuñez G. Function of Nod-like receptors in microbial recognition and host defense. Vol. 227, *Immunological Reviews.* 2009. p. 106–28.

[147] Kim YK, Shin JS, Nahm MH. NOD-like receptors in infection, immunity, and diseases. Vol. 57, *Yonsei Medical Journal.* Yonsei University College of Medicine; 2016. p. 5–14.

[148] Lai CH, Wang KC, Lee FT, Tsai HW, Ma CY, Cheng TL, et al. Toll-like receptor 4 is essential in the development of abdominal aortic aneurysm. *PLoS One*. 2016 Jan 7;11(1).

[149] Gao W, Xiong Y, Li Q, Yang H. Inhibition of toll-like receptor signaling as a promising therapy for inflammatory diseases: A journey from molecular to nano therapeutics. Vol. 8, *Frontiers in Physiology*. Frontiers Media S.A.; 2017.

[150] Wu D, Ren P, Zheng Y, Zhang L, Xu G, Xie W, et al. NLRP3-caspase-1 inflammasome degrades contractile proteins implications for aortic biomechanical dysfunction and aneurysm and dissection formation. *Arterioscler Thromb Vasc Biol*. 2017;37(4):694–706.

[151] Roberts RL, Van Rij AM, Phillips LV, Young S, McCormick SPA, Merriman TR, et al. Interaction of the inflammasome genes CARD8 and NLRP3 in abdominal aortic aneurysms. *Atherosclerosis*. 2011 Sep;218(1):123–6.

[152] Charles A Janeway J, Travers P, Walport M, Shlomchik MJ. The major histocompatibility complex and its functions. Garland Science; 2001. Arakama M-H, Eleanor P. Pamugas G, A. Danguilan R. The impact of HLA-ABDR mismatch on acute rejection and graft function among Filipino kidney transplant recipients. *Trends Transplant*. 2017;10(3).

[153] I. Arakama M-H, Eleanor P. Pamugas G, A. Danguilan R. The impact of HLA-ABDR mismatch on acute rejection and graft function among Filipino kidney transplant recipients. *Trends Transplant*. 2017;10(3).

[154] Noble JA, Valdes AM. Genetics of the HLA region in the prediction of type 1 diabetes. *Curr Diab Rep*. 2011 Dec;11(6):533–42.

[155] Chen B, Li J, He C, Li D, Tong W, Zou Y, et al. Role of HLA-B27 in the pathogenesis of ankylosing spondylitis (Review). *Mol Med Rep*. 2017 Apr 1;15(4):1943–51.

[156] Nepom GT. Major histocompatibility complex-directed susceptibility to rheumatoid arthritis. Vol. 68, *Advances in Immunology*. Academic Press Inc.; 1998. p. 315–32.

[157] Moñux G, Serrano FJ, Vigil P, De la Concha EG. Role of HLA-DR in the pathogenesis of abdominal aortic aneurysm. *Eur J Vasc Endovasc Surg.* 2003 Aug 1;26(2):211–4.

[158] Anaya-Ayala JE, Hernandez-Doño S, Escamilla-Tilch M, Marquez-Garcia J, Hernandez-Sotelo K, Lozano-Corona R, et al. Genetic polymorphism of HLA-DRB1 alleles in Mexican mestizo patients with abdominal aortic aneurysms. *BMC Med Genet.* 2019 Jun 7;20(1).

[159] Ogata T, Gregoire L, Goddard KAB, Skunca M, Tromp G, Lancaster WD, et al. Evidence for association between the HLA-DQA locus and abdominal aortic aneurysms in the Belgian population: A case control study. *BMC Med Genet.* 2006 Jul 31;7.

[160] Redondo MJ, Fain PR, Eisenbarth GS. Genetics of type 1A diabetes. Vol. 56, *Recent Progress in Hormone Research*. Endocrine Society; 2001. p. 69–89.

[161] Marchini M, Antonioli R, Lleò A, Barili M, Caronni M, Origgi L, et al. HLA class II antigens associated with lupus nephritis in Italian SLE patients. *Hum Immunol.* 2003 Apr 1;64(4):462–8.

[162] Haveman JW, van den Berg AP, Verhoeven ELG, Nijsten MWN, van den Dungen JJAM, The TH, et al. HLA-DR expression on monocytes and systemic inflammation in patients with ruptured abdominal aortic aneurysms. *Crit Care.* 2006 Aug 9;10(4).

[163] Krummel MF, Allison JP. CD28 and CTLA-4 have opposing effects on the response of T ceils to stimulation. *J Exp Med.* 1995 Aug 1;182(2):459–65.

[164] Hebbar M, Jeannin P, Magistrelli G, Hatron PY, Hachulla E, Devulder B, et al. Detection of circulating soluble CD28 in patients with systemic lupus erythematosus, primary Sjögren's syndrome and systemic sclerosis. *Clin Exp Immunol.* 2004;136(2):388–92.

[165] Weyand CM, Berry GJ, Goronzy JJ. The immunoinhibitory PD-1/PD-L1 pathway in inflammatory blood vessel disease. *J Leukoc Biol.* 2017 Aug 28;jlb.3MA0717-283.

[166] Sakthivel P, Shively V, Kakoulidou M, Pearce W, Lefvert AK. The soluble forms of CD28, CD86 and CTLA-4 constitute possible

immunological markers in patients with abdominal aortic aneurysm. *J Intern Med.* 2007 Apr;261(4):399–407.

[167] Wong CK, Lit LCW, Tam LS, Li EK, Lam CWK. Aberrant production of soluble costimulatory molecules CTLA-4, CD28, CD80 and CD86 in patients with systemic lupus erythematosus. *Rheumatology.* 2005 Aug;44(8):989–94.

[168] Ip WK, Wong CK, Leung TF, Lam CWK. Elevation of plasma soluble T cell costimulatory molecules CTLA-4, CD28 and CD80 in children with allergic asthma. *Int Arch Allergy Immunol.* 2005 May;137(1):45–52.

[169] Wang XB, Kakoulidou M, Giscombe R, Qiu Q, Huang DR, Pirskanen R, et al. Abnormal expression of CTLA-4 by T cells from patients with myasthenia gravis: Effect of an AT-rich gene sequence. *J Neuroimmunol.* 2002 Sep;130(1–2):224–32.

[170] Oaks MK, Hallett KM, Penwell RT, Stauber EC, Warren SJ, Tector AJ. A native soluble form of CTLA-4. *Cell Immunol.* 2000 May 1;201(2):144–53.

[171] Bour-Jordan H, Esensten JH, Martinez-Llordella M, Penaranda C, Stumpf M, Bluestone JA. Intrinsic and extrinsic control of peripheral T-cell tolerance by costimulatory molecules of the CD28/B7 family. Vol. 241, *Immunological Reviews.* 2011. p. 180–205.

[172] Avina-Zubieta JA, Thomas J, Sadatsafavi M, Lehman AJ, Lacaille D. Risk of incident cardiovascular events in patients with rheumatoid arthritis: A meta-analysis of observational studies. *Ann Rheum Dis.* 2012 Sep;71(9):1524–9.

[173] Shovman O, Tiosano S, Comaneshter D, Cohen AD, Amital H, Sherf M. Aortic aneurysm associated with rheumatoid arthritis: a population-based cross-sectional study. *Clin Rheumatol.* 2016 Nov 1;35(11):2657–61.

[174] Kang EH, Jin Y, Brill G, Lewey J, Patorno E, Desai RJ, et al. Comparative cardiovascular risk of abatacept and tumor necrosis factor inhibitors in patients with rheumatoid arthritis with and without diabetes mellitus: A multidatabase cohort study. *J Am Heart Assoc.* 2018 Feb 1;7(3).

[175] Zhang H, Watanabe R, Berry GJ, Vaglio A, Liao YJ, Warrington KJ, et al. Immunoinhibitory checkpoint deficiency in medium & large vessel vasculitis. *Proc Natl Acad Sci U S A*. 2017 Feb 7;114(6):E970–9.

[176] Gotsman I, Grabie N, Dacosta R, Sukhova G, Sharpe A, Lichtman AH. Proatherogenic immune responses are regulated by the PD-1/PD-L pathway in mice. *J Clin Invest*. 2007 Oct 1;117(10):2974–82.

[177] Ito S, Ansari P, Sakatsume M, Dickensheets H, Vazquez N, Donnelly RP, et al. Interleukin-10 Inhibits Expression of Both Interferon □– and Interferon γ– Induced Genes by Suppressing Tyrosine Phosphorylation of STAT1. *Blood* [Internet]. 1999 Mar 1;93(5):1456–63. Available from: https://ashpublications.org/blood/article/93/5/1456/247850/Interleukin10-Inhibits-Expression-of-Both

[178] Abbas AK, Murphy KM, Sher A. Functional diversity of helper T lymphocytes. Vol. 383, *Nature*. 1996. p. 787–93.

[179] Xiong W, MacTaggart J, Knispel R, Worth J, Persidsky Y, Baxter BT. Blocking TNF-α Attenuates Aneurysm Formation in a Murine Model. *J Immunol*. 2009 Aug 15;183(4):2741–6.

[180] Gu J, Hu J, Zhang H, Xiao Z, Fang Z, Qian H, et al. Time-dependent changes of plasma inflammatory biomarkers in type A aortic dissection patients without optimal medical management. *J Cardiothorac Surg* [Internet]. 2015 Dec 16;10(1):3. Available from: http://cardiothoracicsurgery.biomedcentral.com/articles/10.1186/s13019-014-0199-0

[181] Batra R, Suh MK, Carson JS, Dale MA, Meisinger TM, Fitzgerald M, et al. IL-1β (Interleukin-1β) and TNF-α (Tumor Necrosis Factor-α) Impact Abdominal Aortic Aneurysm Formation by Differential Effects on Macrophage Polarization. *Arterioscler Thromb Vasc Biol* [Internet]. 2018;38(2):457–63. Available from: http://www.ncbi.nlm.nih.gov/pubmed/29217508

[182] Maini RN, Elliott MJ, Charles PJ, Feldmann M. Immunological intervention reveals reciprocal roles for tumor necrosis factor-α and interleukin-10 in rheumatoid arthritis and systemic lupus

erythematosus. *Springer Semin Immunopathol.* 1994 Dec;16(2–3):327–36.

[183] Vilček J, Feldmann M. Historical review: Cytokines as therapeutics and targets of therapeutics. Vol. 25, *Trends in Pharmacological Sciences.* 2004. p. 201–9.

[184] Feldmann M. Development of anti-TNF therapy for rheumatoid arthritis. Vol. 2, *Nature Reviews Immunology.* European Association for Cardio-Thoracic Surgery; 2002. p. 364–71.

[185] Habashi JP, Judge DP, Holm TM, Cohn RD, Loeys BL, Cooper TK, et al. Losartan, an AT1 antagonist, prevents aortic aneurysm in a mouse model of Marfan syndrome. *Science* (80-). 2006 Apr 7;312(5770):117–21.

[186] Chen X, Lu H, Rateri DL, Cassis LA, Daugherty A. Conundrum of angiotensin II and TGF-β interactions in aortic aneurysms. Vol. 13, *Current Opinion in Pharmacology.* 2013. p. 180–5.

[187] Takeda N, Hara H, Fujiwara T, Kanaya T, Maemura S, Komuro I. TGF-β Signaling-Related Genes and Thoracic Aortic Aneurysms and Dissections. *Int J Mol Sci* [Internet]. 2018 Jul 21;19(7). Available from: http://www.ncbi.nlm.nih.gov/pubmed/30037098

[188] Wang Y, Yin P, Chen Y-H, Yu Y-S, Ye W-X, Huang H-Y, et al. A functional variant of SMAD4 enhances macrophage recruitment and inflammatory response via TGF-β signal activation in Thoracic aortic aneurysm and dissection. *Aging* (Albany NY) [Internet]. 2018;10(12):3683–701. Available from: http://www.ncbi.nlm.nih.gov/pubmed/30530919

[189] Yang P, Schmit BM, Fu C, DeSart K, Oh SP, Berceli SA, et al. Smooth muscle cell-specific Tgfbr1 deficiency promotes aortic aneurysm formation by stimulating multiple signaling events. *Sci Rep* [Internet]. 2016 Dec 14;6(1):35444. Available from: http://www.nature.com/articles/srep35444

[190] Zeng L, Dang TA, Schunkert H. *Genetics links between transforming growth factor β pathway and coronary disease* [Internet]. Atherosclerosis Elsevier Ireland Ltd; Oct 1, 2016 p. 237–46. Available from: http://www.ncbi.nlm.nih.gov/pubmed/27596813

[191] Benke K, Ágg B, Szilveszter B, Tarr F, Nagy ZB, Pólos M, et al. The role of transforming growth factor-beta in Marfan syndrome. Vol. 20, *Cardiology Journal*. 2013. p. 227–34.

[192] Bertoli-Avella AM, Gillis E, Morisaki H, Verhagen JMAA, de Graaf BM, van de Beek G, et al. Mutations in a TGF-β Ligand, TGFB3, Cause Syndromic Aortic Aneurysms and Dissections. *J Am Coll Cardiol* [Internet]. 2015 Apr 7;65(13):1324–36. Available from: http://www.ncbi.nlm.nih.gov/pubmed/25835445

[193] Doyle AJ, Redmond EM, Gillespie DL, Knight PA, Cullen JP, Cahill PA, et al. *Differential Expression of Hedgehog/Notch and Transforming Growth Factor-β in Human Abdominal Aortic Aneurysms* [Internet]. Aug 1, 2015. Available from: http://www.ncbi.nlm.nih.gov/pubmed/24768363

[194] Wu D, Shen YH, Russell L, Coselli JS, LeMaire SA. Molecular mechanisms of thoracic aortic dissection. *J Surg Res* [Internet]. 2013 Oct;184(2):907–24. Available from: http://www.ncbi.nlm.nih.gov/pubmed/23856125

[195] Angelov SN, Hu JH, Wei H, Airhart N, Shi M, Dichek DA, et al. TGF-β (Transforming Growth Factor-β) Signaling Protects the Thoracic and Abdominal Aorta From Angiotensin II-Induced Pathology by Distinct Mechanisms. *Arterioscler Thromb Vasc Biol* [Internet]. 2017 Nov;37(11):2102–13. Available from: https://www.ahajournals.org/doi/10.1161/ATVBAHA.117.309401

[196] Wei H, Hu JH, Angelov SN, Fox K, Yan J, Enstrom R, et al. Aortopathy in a Mouse Model of Marfan Syndrome Is Not Mediated by Altered Transforming Growth Factor β Signaling. *J Am Heart Assoc* [Internet]. 2017 Jan 24;6(1). Available from: http://www.ncbi.nlm.nih.gov/pubmed/28119285

[197] Theruvath TP, Jones JA, Ikonomidis JS. Matrix metalloproteinases and descending aortic aneurysms: parity, disparity, and switch [Internet]. *Journal of Cardiac Surgery NIH Public Access*; Jan, 2012 p. 81–90. Available from: http://www.ncbi.nlm.nih.gov/pubmed/21958052

[198] Rundhaug JE. Matrix metalloproteinases and angiogenesis. Vol. 9, *Journal of cellular and molecular medicine*. 2005. p. 267–85.

[199] Gialeli C, Theocharis AD, Karamanos NK. Roles of matrix metalloproteinases in cancer progression and their pharmacological targeting. Vol. 278, *FEBS Journal*. 2011. p. 16–27.

[200] Liu P, Sun M, Sader S. Matrix metalloproteinases in cardiovascular disease. *Can J Cardiol*. 2006;22(SUPPL. B):25B-30B.

[201] Ikonomidis JS, Gibson WC, Butler JE, McClister DM, Sweterlitsch SE, Thompson RP, et al. Effects of deletion of the tissue inhibitor of matrix metalloproteinases-1 gene on the progression of murine thoracic aortic aneurysms. *Circulation*. 2004 Sep 14;110(11 SUPPL.).

[202] Tamarina NA, McMillan WD, Shively VP, Pearce WH. Expression of matrix metalloproteinases and their inhibitors in aneurysms and normal aorta. In: *Surgery*. Mosby Inc.; 1997. p. 264–72.

[203] Maguire EM, Pearce SWA, Xiao R, Oo AY, Xiao Q. Matrix metalloproteinase in abdominal aortic aneurysm and aortic dissection. Vol. 12, *Pharmaceuticals*. MDPI AG; 2019.

[204] Ikonomidis JS, Jones JA, Barbour JR, Stroud RE, Clark LL, Kaplan BS, et al. Expression of matrix metalloproteinases and endogenous inhibitors within ascending aortic aneurysms of patients with bicuspid or tricuspid aortic valves. *J Thorac Cardiovasc Surg*. 2007 Apr;133(4):1028–36.

[205] Zervoudaki A, Economou E, Stefanadis C, Pitsavos C, Tsioufis K, Aggeli C, et al. Plasma levels of active extracellular matrix metalloproteinases 2 and 9 in patients with essential hypertension before and after antihypertensive treatment. *J Hum Hypertens*. 2003 Feb 1;17(2):119–24.

[206] Yu Q, Stamenkovic I. Cell surface-localized matrix metalloproteinase-9 proteolytically activates TGF-β and promotes tumor invasion and angiogenesis. *Genes Dev*. 2000 Jan 15;14(2):163–76.

[207] Davis V, Persidskaia R, Baca-Regen L, Itoh Y, Nagase H, Persidsky Y, et al. Matrix metalloproteinase-2 production and its binding to the

matrix are increased in abdominal aortic aneurysms. *Arterioscler Thromb Vasc Biol.* 1998;18(10):1625–33.

[208] Zhang X, Shen YH, LeMaire SA. Thoracic aortic dissection: Are matrix metalloproteinases involved? Vol. 17, *Vascular.* 2009. p. 147–57.

[209] Shen M, Lee J, Basu R, Sakamuri SSVP, Wang X, Fan D, et al. Divergent roles of matrix metalloproteinase 2 in pathogenesis of thoracic aortic aneurysm. *Arterioscler Thromb Vasc Biol.* 2015 Apr 27;35(4):888–98.

[210] Barbour JR, Stroud RE, Lowry AS, Clark LL, Leone AM, Jones JA, et al. Temporal disparity in the induction of matrix metalloproteinases and tissue inhibitors of metalloproteinases after thoracic aortic aneurysm formation. *J Thorac Cardiovasc Surg.* 2006 Oct; 132(4):788–95.

[211] Prasad K, Sarkar A, Zafar MA, Shoker A, Moselhi HE, Tranquilli M, et al. Advanced Glycation End Products and its Soluble Receptors in the Pathogenesis of Thoracic Aortic Aneurysm. *Aorta (Stamford, Conn)* [Internet]. 2016 Feb;4(1):1–10. Available from: http://www.ncbi.nlm.nih.gov/pubmed/27766267

[212] Barbour JR, Spinale FG, Ikonomidis JS. Proteinase Systems and Thoracic Aortic Aneurysm Progression. Vol. 139, *Journal of Surgical Research.* 2007. p. 292–307.

[213] Liu C, Zhang C, Jia L, Chen B, Liu L, Sun J, et al. Interleukin-3 stimulates matrix metalloproteinase 12 production from macrophages promoting thoracic aortic aneurysm/dissection. *Clin Sci (Lond)* [Internet]. 2018 Mar 30;132(6):655–68. Available from: http://www.ncbi.nlm.nih.gov/pubmed/29523595

[214] Xiong W, Mactaggart J, Knispel R, Worth J, Zhu Z, Li Y, et al. Inhibition of reactive oxygen species attenuates aneurysm formation in a murine model. *Atherosclerosis.* 2009 Jan;202(1):128–34.

[215] Luo F, Zhou X-LL, Li J-JJ, Hui R-TT. Inflammatory response is associated with aortic dissection. [Internet]. *Ageing Research Reviews* Jan, 2009 p. 31–5. Available from: http://www.ncbi.nlm.nih.gov/pubmed/18789403

[216] Görlach A, Bertram K, Hudecova S, Krizanova O. Calcium and ROS: A mutual interplay. Vol. 6, *Redox Biology*. Elsevier B.V.; 2015. p. 260–71.

[217] Meli DN, Christen S, Leib SL. Matrix Metalloproteinase-9 in Pneumococcal Meningitis: Activation via an Oxidative Pathway. *J Infect Dis* [Internet]. 2003 May;187(9):1411–5. Available from: https://academic.oup.com/jid/article-lookup/doi/10.1086/374644

[218] Rajagopalan S, Meng XP, Ramasamy S, Harrison DG, Galis ZS. Reactive oxygen species produced by macrophage-derived foam cells regulate the activity of vascular matrix metalloproteinases in vitro: Implications for atherosclerotic plaque stability. *J Clin Invest*. 1996 Dec 1;98(11):2572–9.

[219] Zhang J, Schmidt J, Ryschich E, Mueller-Schilling M, Schumacher H, Allenberg JR. Inducible nitric oxide synthase is present in human abdominal aortic aneurysm and promotes oxidative vascular injury. *J Vasc Surg*. 2003;38(2):360–7.

[220] Johanning JM, Franklin DP, Han DC, Carey DJ, Elmore JR. Inhibition of inducible nitric oxide synthase limits nitric oxide production and experimental aneurysm expansion. *J Vasc Surg*. 2001;33(3):579–86.

[221] Lizarbe TR, Tarín C, Gómez M, Lavin B, Aracil E, Orte LM, et al. Nitric oxide induces the progression of abdominal aortic aneurysms through the matrix metalloproteinase inducer EMMPRIN. *Am J Pathol*. 2009;175(4):1421–30.

[222] Allen-Redpath K, Aldrovandi M, Lauder SN, Gketsopoulou A, Tyrrell VJ, Slatter DA, et al. Phospholipid membranes drive abdominal aortic aneurysm development through stimulating coagulation factor activity. *Proc Natl Acad Sci U S A*. 2019 Apr 16;116(16):8038–47.

[223] Hinterseher I, Erdman R, Donoso LA, Vrabec TR, Schworer CM, Lillvis JH, et al. Role of complement cascade in abdominal aortic aneurysms. *Arterioscler Thromb Vasc Biol*. 2011 Jul;31(7):1653–60.

[224] Capella JF, Paik DC, Yin NX, Gervasoni JE, Tilson MD. Complement activation and subclassification of tissue immunoglobulin G in the abdominal aortic aneurysm. *J Surg Res*. 1996;65(1):31–3.

[225] Pagano MB, Zhou HF, Ennis TL, Wu X, Lambris JD, Atkinson JP, et al. Complement-dependent neutrophil recruitment is critical for the development of elastase-induced abdominal aortic aneurysm. *Circulation*. 2009 Apr 7;119(13):1805–13.

[226] Bradley DT, Badger SA, Bown MJ, Sayers RD, Hughes AE. Coding polymorphisms in the genes of the alternative complement pathway and abdominal aortic aneurysm. *Int J Immunogenet*. 2011 Jun;38(3):243–8.

[227] Roccabianca S, Ateshian GA, Humphrey JD. Biomechanical roles of medial pooling of glycosaminoglycans in thoracic aortic dissection. *Biomech Model Mechanobiol* [Internet]. 2014 Jan;13(1):13–25. Available from: http://www.ncbi.nlm.nih.gov/pubmed/23494585

[228] Humphrey JDD. Possible mechanical roles of glycosaminoglycans in thoracic aortic dissection and associations with dysregulated transforming growth factor-β. *J Vasc Res* [Internet]. 2013 Dec;50(1):1–10. Available from: http://www.ncbi.nlm.nih.gov/pubmed/23018968

[229] Roccabianca S, Bellini C, Humphrey JD. Computational modelling suggests good, bad and ugly roles of glycosaminoglycans in arterial wall mechanics and mechanobiology. *J R Soc Interface* [Internet]. 2014 Aug 6;11(97):20140397. Available from: http://www.ncbi.nlm.nih.gov/pubmed/24920112

[230] Cikach FS, Koch CD, Mead TJ, Galatioto J, Willard BB, Emerton KB, et al. Massive Aggrecan and Versican Accumulation in Thoracic Aortic Aneurysm and Dissection. *JCI insight* [Internet]. 2018 Mar 8;3(5). Available from: http://www.ncbi.nlm.nih.gov/pubmed/29515038

[231] Borges LF, Touat Z, Leclercq A, Al Haj Zen A, Jondeau' G, Franc B, et al. Tissue diffusion and retention of metalloproteinases in ascending aortic aneurysms and dissections. *Hum Pathol*. 2009 Mar;40(3):306–13.

[232] Wight TN. Arterial remodeling in vascular disease: A key role for hyaluronan and versican. Vol. 13, *Frontiers in Bioscience*. 2008. p. 4933–7.

[233] Ahmadzadeh H, Rausch MK, Humphrey JD. Modeling lamellar disruption within the aortic wall using a particle-based approach. *Sci Rep.* 2019 Dec 1;9(1).

In: Aortic Aneurysms
Editor: Amer Harky

ISBN: 978-1-53617-677-3
© 2020 Nova Science Publishers, Inc.

Chapter 2

ENDOVASCULAR STENT GRAFTING OF THORACIC AORTIC ANEURYSM

Chi Wei Ong[1], Foad Kabinejadian[2], Ala Elhelali[3] and Hwa Liang Leo[1],*

[1]Department of Biomedical Engineering,
National University of Singapore, Singapore
[2]Department of Biomedical Engineering, Tulane University,
New Orleans, LA, US
[3]Department of Plastic and Reconstructive Surgery, Johns Hopkins
University, Baltimore, MD, US

ABSTRACT

Thoracic aortic aneurysm (TAA) can be a silent killer if left untreated. Open surgery needs a longer recovery process and is not suitable for high-risk patients. Thoracic endovascular aortic repair (TEVAR) has been introduced as a less invasive approach to management of thoracic aortic aneurysm (TAA). Common TEVAR approaches involve implantation of a simple Dacron stent graft through a catheter. However, the effectiveness of

---

* Corresponding Author's Email: bielhl@nus.edu.sg.

TEVAR in the management of TAA is often limited by the complex anatomy of the aortic arch. Branched and fenestrated stent grafts have been developed to preserve perfusion of superior branches with a low incidence of sealing zone failure. The disadvantage of the branched and fenestrated techniques is that they require custom-made devices and complex procedures, which make them less promising in urgent TEVAR. Moreover, the branched and fenestrated stent grafts have been shown to be prone to proximal endoleak that could lead to increased mortality. Another novel technique is called chimney technique. Chimney technique is a stent placed parallel to the aortic stent graft to preserve the blood flow to superior branches that was overstented to achieve an adequate seal. Even though the technique outcome is encouraging, it is difficult to fabricate a dedicated covered stent for chimney repair.

In this chapter, we will discuss the novel stenting technique for TAA which applies engineering fluid mechanics knowledge on the innovation of medical device. Innovative devices such as the multilayer flow modulator (MFM) have recently been proposed to provide an alternative endovascular treatment. The main purpose of MFM is to decrease the risk of rupture by modulating the flow pattern which can then lead to a reduction in local shear stress along the weakened artery wall. We will evaluate the pros and cons of disruptive technologies such as MFM and compare them with the above-mentioned methods such as conventional TEVAR, fenestrated, and chimney repair. An overview of the elective and emergency approach using MFM and other innovative approaches published in the existing literature will be discussed. This review indicates that although most of the innovative techniques appear to be successful, the expansion of aneurysm does not slow down immediately, and usually, only a short period of follow up results are presented. These innovations will require more clinical trials and longer follow up studies to confirm the feasibility of this disruptive technology. The presented review in this chapter can provide great insight into the nature, diagnosis, and potential improvements for the intervention involving TAA.

Keywords: multilayer stent, MFM, TEVAR, TAA, aneurysm

INTRODUCTION

Since 2008 when Henry et al. (Henry et al. 2008) reported the first results of the multilayer flow modular (MFM) stent to treat the aortic aneurysm, this treatment approach has caught attention of health care professionals as an alternative for treating complex aortic aneurysm especially those with more than one side branches (Stefanov et al. 2016). However, the success of multilayer flow modulator (MFM) depends on appropriate anatomic criteria and proper surgical planning (Sherif Sultan et al. 2017, Sultan, Hynes, and Sultan 2014). As suggested by the literature, MFM is not a perfect solution for patients who lived in borrow times and should not be used in patients in whom no other treatment option are feasible (Sultan, Hynes, and Sultan 2014). Furthermore, some cases have shown that MFM cannot stop the aneurysm from further growth immediately after repair, but long-term effects of the device have not yet to be tested with large clinical trials. Since the first suggested guideline provided by Sultan et al. (Sultan, Hynes, and Sultan 2014) in 2014, there have been clinical trials and several publications ongoing from 2015-2019 to test the feasibility of multilayer flow modulator for treating the aortic disease, e.g., abdominal aortic aneurysm, complex thoracoabdominal aneurysm, and dissection (Costache et al. 2018, Hynes et al. 2016, Vaislic et al. 2016, Benjelloun et al. 2016, Ovalı and Sevin 2018b, Rikhtegar Nezami et al. 2018, Tirziu et al. 2018, Ucci et al. 2018, Spinella et al. 2018, Schafigh et al. 2018, Zhang et al. 2014, Zeng, Huang, and He 2016, Ong et al. 2019, Cavalcante et al. 2015, Lowe et al. 2016). This innovative concept of turning the turbulent flow into laminar to lessen the wall stress exerted on the aneurysmal wall inspires a series of innovative design to treat the aneurysm which will be discussed in later sections.

PREVALENCE OF AORTIC ANEURYSM

Despite significant advancements in clinical care and treatment, cardiovascular disease is still the leading cause of mortality and morbidity in developed and developing countries (Mozaffarian et al. 2016). One type of cardiovascular disease that remains a challenge is aortic aneurysm. It is the primary cause of 9,863 deaths in 2014 and a secondary cause of more than 17,215 deaths in the United States in 2009.

KNOWN TREATMENT

Treatments for aortic aneurysms can generally be categorized into open surgery and thoracic endovascular aneurysm repair (TEVAR). For the past few decades, the open-chest-approach remains the major surgical treatment for TAAs. However, due to its invasive nature and the long recovery time required, open-chest surgery is associated with high mortality and morbidity rates (Harvard 2010). A relatively less-invasive method, TEVAR is recognized as an alternative. Both methods are discussed in the following sections.

Open Surgery

Conventional surgery for TAAs can repair or replace the TAA through a procedure called an open thoracic aortic aneurysm repair. It begins with an incision along the side of the chest with the assistance of a special surgical tool to prevent the blood flow in the aorta above and below an aneurysm. Once the incision is complete, the part of aorta with the aneurysm is replaced with a Dacron graft. The graft is sewn in place with fine stitches, and the incision is sealed. The size of the incision can vary, depending on the size of the aneurysm. Most patients have extensive length of intensive care unit (ICU) stay postoperative ranging from 7–10 days (Eagleton 2004). Open surgical repair is associated with substantial perioperative risk such as cardiac morbidity, pneumonia, and renal mobility (Elkouri et al. 2004). However, a recent study showed that although open surgical repair has risk of complication, it can bring more benefit to the younger patients with long life expectancy and low-perioperative risk and remain an essential treatment modality in many circumstances such as unfavorable anatomy for endovascular repair or connective tissue disorder (Swerdlow, Wu, and Schermerhorn 2019).

Hybrid Repair

For complex aortic aneurysms, such as thoracoabdominal aortic aneurysm (TAAA), there is another type of surgical intervention, namely a hybrid repair. This surgery poses a medium risk compared to the high-risk open-chest repair since it can reduce the burden of the procedure and reduce the aneurysm thrombosis caused by the extensive surgical procedure done in an open chest surgery. Hybrid TAAA repair was originally introduced by Quinones-Baldrich and colleagues (Quiñones-Baldrich et al. 1999) as an alternative to open repair. Its advantage included avoiding aortic cross-clamping, thoracotomy, single-lung ventilation, and prolonged ischemia. Hybrid repair generally involves 1 or 2 stages which involve both open surgery and endovascular repair. In two-stage hybrid repair approach, aortic visceral branches are rerouted with 8- or 10-mm bypass grafts with aortic reattachment sites above or below the proposed endovascular zone, followed by endovascular exclusion of the aneurysm, which then covers the vessel origins (Orozco-Sevilla, Weldon, and Coselli 2018). Hybrid repair has always been thought only suitable for high-risk surgical patients and in patients with anatomy unfit for endovascular repair (Tshomba et al. 2012). However, a recent study showed that hybrid repair seems to be an effective and safe procedure for treatment of arch aortic aneurysm (Yoshitake et al. 2019); and it appears to be durable at a mid-term follow up (Bishry and Krebber 2019, Yoshitake et al. 2019). Hence, it has the potential to be an effective treatment for aortic arch aneurysm.

Thoracic Endovascular Aneurysm Repair (TEVAR)

Since the first homograft repair of a TAA reported by (Swan et al. 1950) and (De Bakey and Cooley 1953), TEVAR was the first alternative treatment proposed for open surgery in treating TAA (Mitchell et al. 1996). Open surgery is often accompanied by excessive risks such as high mortality rates, as well as disabling complications such as permanent paraplegia or stroke in patients who survive (Jonker et al. 2011). In contrast, TEVAR is relatively safer compared to open surgery, since it demonstrates better perioperative results and achieves a similar long-term outcome as open surgical repair, e.g., an aneurysm is well-sealed by the stent graft. Recent reports have shown that TEVAR is more desirable as a less invasive treatment for aortic aneurysm (Lioupis and Abraham 2011, Rolph et al. 2013). A nonrandomized study revealed that TEVAR may cut down the risk of premature death, cardiac complications and period of stay in the hospital, compared to open chest surgery (Cheng et al. 2010). Common TEVAR approaches involve the implantation of a Dacron stent graft, fenestrated endograft, and chimney repair (Kasemi et al. 2015).

Branched and Fenestrated Stent Grafts

To provide optimal sealing to a TAA, fenestrated stent grafts have been developed to preserve perfusion of the superior branches to reduce the failure of sealing zone. The first application of a fenestrated stent graft was published in 1999 (Browne et al. 1999) after a seminar report was written by Parodi (Parodi, Palmaz, and Barone 1991) on the use of an endograft for the repair of an abdominal aortic aneurysm (AAA). Since then, the capability of fenestrated stent grafts in shifting the seal zone to a higher position in the aorta has accelerated the evolution of the fenestrated technique (Scurr and McWilliams 2007).

Beside the fenestrated stent graft, a branched stent graft was designed for aneurysms that involve vital aortic side branches such as supra-renal arteries, Type 4 thoracoabdominal aneurysms, or aortic arch aneurysms. The difference between the branched stent graft and the fenestrated stent graft is that the branched stent graft is already attached to the body of the endograft and deploys itself into aortic branches, rather than premade windows for aortic branches such as in the fenestrated graft. Therefore, the branch of the stent graft can close the gap between the stent graft and the native aortic wall, which in turn preserves perfusion of the aortic side branch for optimal sealing (Kasipandian and Pichel 2012).

The disadvantage of the branch and fenestrated techniques is that they need custom-made devices and complicated surgical procedures, which make them less feasible for emergency cases. Moreover, the branched and fenestrated stent grafts are prone to proximal endoleak that could lead to higher mortality rate (O'Callaghan et al. 2015).

Chimney Repair

Another novel repair technique is called the chimney technique. The first reported case using the chimney technique was in the salvage of unintentionally over-stented branch vessels during endovascular repair in 2003 (Greenberg et al. 2003). The chimney technique is named after its deployment method. During the chimney repair approach, the proximal parts of second stent that is deployed from the supra-aortic branches is placed parallel to the main aortic stent graft, preserving the blood flow to the overstented superior branches, in order to achieve an adequate seal. The purpose of using the chimney graft technique is to prolong the sealing zone of the aortic stent graft by deploying a vital aortic side branch parallel to the main aortic stent graft (Ohrlander et al. 2008). It requires the placement of single or multiple uncovered and covered stents parallel, to the main aortic stent graft to maintain patency of the side branch (Patel et al. 2013). Ideally, a good conformability should be formed between the main stent graft, chimney graft, and the aortic wall. Unfortunately, it does not function perfectly, given that a potential gap found between the main graft and the chimney graft will often result in type I endoleaks that may be due to the unpredictable position of the chimney graft. Even though the outcome of this technique is supportive, it is difficult to manufacture a dedicated covered stent for chimney repair (Lindblad et al. 2015). There are different types of endoleaks still present under different TEVAR techniques. Therefore, a new stent graft design is needed to acknowledge these complications for a better treatment plan.

INNOVATIVE TREATMENTS

Multilayer Flow Modulator

Innovative medical devices such as the multilayer flow modulator (MFM) (Sultan, Hynes, et al. 2014) have recently been proposed to provide an alternative endovascular treatment. The aortic MFM technology was first developed in 2009 for peripheral arteries, followed by a design for an aortic device in 2011 (Cardiatis 2009).

MFM device is a self-expanding device constructed of cobalt alloy wires interconnected in five layers, as shown in Figure 1. It is a flexible device with high kinking and fatigue resistance (Sultan and Hynes 2013, Zeng, Huang, and He 2016). This device is taught to physiologically remodel and heal the aortic aneurysm while preserving branching vessel patency by laminating the blood flow and directing blood flow to the branching vessels. In addition, the MFM reduces the risk of rupture by modulating the flow pattern, inducing favorable blood flow patterns within the aneurysm sac which can then lead to a reduction of local shear stress along the weakened artery wall (Diethrich 2014, Sultan and Hynes 2013, Benjelloun et al. 2016, Rikhtegar Nezami et al. 2018, Zeng, Huang, and He 2016, Stefanov et al. 2016, Morris et al. 2016, Sultan et al. 2016, Sultan, Kavanagh, et al. 2014). The minimally invasiveness of the stent allowing for negligible impact on the patient's co-morbid status is ideal in high-risk patients with multiple comorbidities.

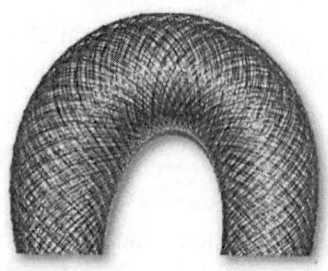

Figure 1. Aortic multilayer flow modulator device.

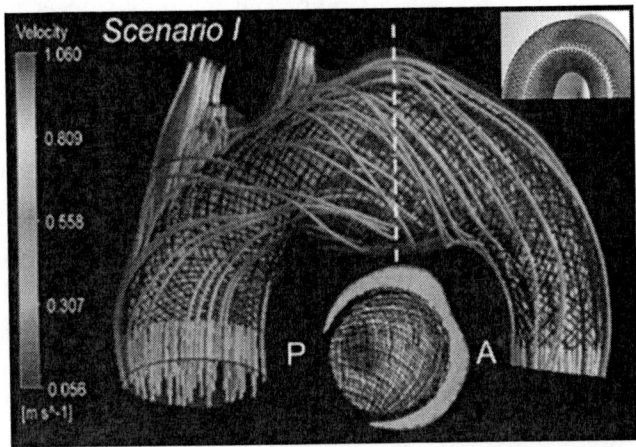

Figure 2. Aneurysm blood flow streamlines and velocity contour. Adopted from with (Stefanov et al. 2016) permission.

Very little experimental work has been conducted on the MFM to assess its performance within the aorta and the aneurysm sac (Stefanov et al. 2016). Stefanov et al. (2016) analysed patient specific rigid walled aneurysm models using computational methods, and reported reduction in wall shear stress with the presence of the MFM and improved pressures and perfusion through the supra-aortic vessels(Stefanov et al. 2016). The results of this study showed that the MFM device promoted organised swirling flow patterns.

The one-year outcome of MFM in the management of thoracoabdominal aortic aneurysms showed a 98.2% technical success rate reported by Sultan and Hynes 2013 (Sultan and Hynes 2013). Although the aneurysm sacs had increased, there were no signs of rupture, and growth of thrombus within the aneurysm sac (Sultan and Hynes 2013). Vaislic et al, 2016 assessed the MFM in thoracoabdominal aneurysm and reported 94.0% all-cause survival at 12 months, and during the 3-year follow-up, seven deaths were reported (Cardiatis 2009). In addition, the low rates of stroke and paraplegia are superior to those of other treatment modalities for similar aortic pathologies (Hynes et al. 2016, Vaislic et al. 2016, Pinto et al. 2017, Kasprzak et al. 2014, Czerny et al. 2012).

Despite the low reported mortality and morbidity rates, it has been reported that the MFM does not perform well in some clinical scenarios (Sultan, Hynes, and Sultan 2014, Debing et al. 2014, Lazaris, Maheras, and Vasdekis 2012). A study by Sultan et al. 2014, reporting on contraindicated cases treated with the MFM. They noted that 10 patients presenting with an aortic rupture all died after MFM implantation. Sultan and colleagues have introduced new recommendations for the use of the MFM (Sherif Sultan et al. 2017). Based on this new instructions for use (IFU), the MFM is not an ideal solution for all cases of throacoabdominal aneurysms, particularly in those with a history of myeloproliferative disorders or coagulation problems, ruptured aortic aneurysms, inadequate arterial access, absence of healthy landing zone, aortic dissection, presence or suspicion of infection, aneurysms with maximum transverse diameter of >6.5 cm or total aneurysm volume >400 cm^3 (Sultan, Hynes, and Sultan 2014, Sherif Sultan et al. 2017, Cavalcante et al. 2015, Lowe et al. 2016). Strictly adhering to the MFM IFU is essential to ensure successful treatment (Sultan, Hynes, and Sultan 2014).

Although the initial testing of MFM looks promising, it undoubtedly also attracts a number of critics from published articles on the feasibility of the device. We have summed up recent evidence of non-randomized controlled trials (RCTs) and RCTs using the MFM between 2016 and 2018 in the following tables (Table 1 and 2).

Based on the data presented in Tables 1 and 2, it appears that the MFM can be an alternative for patients who are unfit for other elective surgical interventions due to complex anatomies. Moreover, for the patients who are high risk and have complicated anatomy, MFM appears to be a good candidate for emergency repair as well since it offers flexibility for fitting different anatomies. However, the long-term outcome for undergoing MFM repair (either elective repair or emergency repair) remains to unveil, and we expect to see more publications and clinical studies on this perspective viewpoint in the future.

Table 1. Summary of MFM application from 2016-2018

Author/Year	Study/objective	Patients with MFM	Methods used	Findings/Conclusion
Costache., 2018 (Costache et al. 2018)	To investigate the effect of Multilayer Flow Modulator (MFM) in the treatment of type B aortic dissection (TBAD) and to present the aortic remodeling using computational fluid dynamics (CFD) analysis over the course of 3-year follow-up.	1	two aortic multilayer stents placed in the compressed true lumen of a hypertensive patient with complicated type B aortic dissection (TBAD)	MFM can help secure the entire aortic wall in the complicated TBAD without blocking flow in the side branches
Hynes 2016 (Hynes et al. 2016)	To evaluate the safety and short-term efficacy of the Streamliner Multilayer Flow Modulator (SMFM) in the management of patients with complex TAAA pathology who are not suitable for alternative interventions in systematic review.	171	a patient-level meta-analysis was conducted to evaluate the aneurysm-related survival in the patient after SMFM implantation.	The SMFM can be implanted in patients with complex anatomy as long as the operators adhere to the Instructions for Use (IFU).
Vaislic, 2016 (Vaislic et al. 2016)	To evaluate midterm outcomes of endovascular repair of types II and III thoracoabdominal aortic aneurysms (TAAA) using the Multilayer Flow Modulator (MFM) in patients who are unfit for open surgery or fenestrated stent-grafts	23	23 patients (mean age 75.8 years; 19 men) with Crawford type II and III TAAA (mean diameter 6.5 cm) were implanted with MFM.	Endovascular repair with the MFM appears to be safe and effective while successfully maintaining branch vessel patency.

Table 1. (Continued)

Author/Year	Study/objective	Patients with MFM	Methods used	Findings/Conclusion
Benjelloun, 2016 (Benjelloun et al. 2016)	To evaluate endovascular repair of thoracoabdominal aortic aneurysms (TAAA) and abdominal aortic aneurysms (AAA) using the Multilayer Flow Modulator (MFM) in high-surgical-risk patients with at least one covered aortic branch	18	18 patients (mean age 61.1 years; 16 men) with TAAA (n = 10, mean diameter 74.4 mm) and AAA (n = 8, mean diameter 67.8 mm) were treated with the MFM	MFM appears to be safe and effective in the treatment of high-surgical-risk TAAA and AAA patients in the mid-term follow up. It can maintain branch vessel patency and reduce the risk of rupture.
Ovali 2018 (Ovali and Sevin 2018b)	Recommend new implantation technique by consider intervening in the extracorporeal circulation and to cut the ascending aorta to perform the surgery	1	Two MFMs (Cardiatis, CTMS 40150) were placed in the aneurysm region for endovascular intervention. The angulation of the MFM stent was corrected manually after the stent was found not reach the targeted region due to complex analysis. Afterward, an MFM stent was implanted aligning from the T4 vertebra level up to the innominate artery distal.	The ascending aorta can be used as an intervention area in the treatment of aortic aneurysms when the endovascular operation cannot be performed due to the difficulty of intervention area or implantation difficulty during operation with MFM implantation

Author/Year	Study/objective	Patients with MFM	Methods used	Findings/Conclusion
Rikhtegrar 2018 (Rikhtegar Nezami et al. 2018)	Examined MFM end-organ perfusion effects by comparing flow in three-dimensional (3-D) arterial models for one patient at pseudohealthy (PH), preintervention (PI), and post-MFM placement (PM) states in a type B aortic dissection (AD)	1	preintervention and post-multilayer flow modulator implantation (PM) geometries from clinical cases of type B AD was constructed and a computational fluid dynamics analysis was performed to examine the flow change before and after intervention.	MFM managed to reduce false lumen blood flow significantly, eliminated local flow disturbances, and globally regulated wall shear stress distribution. It also preserved the physiological perfusion to peripheral vital organs.
Cengiz OvalJ, 2018 (Oval et al. 2018)	Reported early and midterm results of aortic and iliac artery aneurysms treated with MFM	23	23 patients (19 males and 4 females) were treated with MFM stents.	Not all the cases are successful. MFM can be considered as an alternative approach in the treatment of aorta and iliac artery aneurysms including major lateral branches.
Tirziu, 2018 (Tirziu et al. 2018)	Present a retrospective post market series of 14 cases of Penetrating aortic ulcers (PAU) treated with MFM.	14	14 cases of PAU was treated with MFM. Pre- and post-procedure CT angiography and 3D CT reconstructions were used to assess the patency of branch vessels	MFM preserved the patency of all major covered branches without paraplegia, and promoted overall stabilization of treated PAU lesions.

Table 1. (Continued)

Author/Year	Study/objective	Patients with MFM	Methods used	Findings/Conclusion
Ucci, 2018 (Ucci et al. 2018)	Report the outcomes of patients with popliteal artery aneurysm treated with the multilayer flow modulator in three Italian centers.	23	a series of both symptomatic and asymptomatic patients with popliteal artery aneurysm treated with the multilayer flow modulator from 2009 to 2015 was analyzed retrospectivity. Follow up with utlrasound was taken at at 1, 6 and 12 months, and yearly thereafter	Multilayer flow modulator seems a safe option of popliteal artery aneurysms in selected patients.
Walid Ibrahim 2018 (Ibrahim et al. 2018)	reported the early and midterm outcomes of endovascular repair of complex aortic aneurysm cases using MFM in Germany	61	evaluate the mortality and morbidity at 30 days postoperatively for patients abdominal aortic aneurysm (AAA), thoracic aortic aneurysm, or thoracoabdominal aortic aneurysm treated with the MFM in Germany and also assess the freedom from reintervention, rupture and failure model	MFM appears to be technically feasible in treatment of complex aortic aneurysm in terms of mortality and morbidity, with moderate 30-day and acceptable midterm outcomes.

Author/Year	Study/objective	Patients with MFM	Methods used	Findings/Conclusion
Giovanni Spinella, 2018 (Spinella et al. 2018)	Presented the clinical results and aneurysmal sac evolution after MFM placement in patients with TAAA	7	7 patients with TAA was treated with MFM. Thirty-day evaluated outcomes were mortality and complications. Follow-up evaluated outcomes were mortality, aneurysm collateral branches patency, and reintervention	No mortality found in the follow up studies after MFM placement
Ovali & Sevin 2018 (Ovali and Sevin 2018a)	Assess the early and mid-term results of the combined use of MFM and conventional stent grafts in aortic aneurysms and Type B aortic dissections in Turkey	6	Six patients treated with MFM in combination with conventional stent grafts. The patients were followed for the development of any clinical events during 12 months	Multilayer flow modulator stents seem to be safe in the treatment of aortic aneurysms with major side branches. The combined use of stents with different stent-graft devices increase the success rate and reduce the complication rate in complex aortic aneurysms.

Table 1. (Continued)

Author/Year	Study/objective	Patients with MFM	Methods used	Findings/Conclusion
Schafigh, 2018 (Schafigh et al. 2018)	Reported MFM treatment in a patient with progressive chronic type B dissection and contraindication for open surgery	1	a Cardiatis Multilayer Flow Modulator implanted in a patient with progressive chronic type B dissection and contraindication for open surgery with the stented area beginning in the distal ascending aorta and ending approximately 2 cm above the iliacal bifurcation.	A ruptured retrograde type A aortic dissection was found two weeks after the intervention. It is caused by the stent's uncovered proximal ends.
Melnic, 2018 (Melnic et al. 2018)	Assess the results of up to 36-month follow-up after complete coverage of supra-aortic trunks with MFM for complex aortic diseases.	29	29 patients with complex aortic disease underwent endovascular repair with an MFM stent in the prospective study. Computational fluid dynamics analysis was performed at each follow up	MFM stents are safe in the treatment of complex aortic diseases. Total coverage of all supra-aortic trunks does not lead to any neurologic complication

Author/Year	Study/objective	Patients with MFM	Methods used	Findings/Conclusion
Calik, 2018 (Calik and Erkut 2018)	Present a successful endovascular treatment of a Stanford Type A aortic dissection by the MFM in a patient at high risk of surgery.	1	MFM was implanted in a patient with chronic Type A dissection. He has diabetes, hypertension and second degree mitral insufficiency who underwent coronary artery bypass grafting. The proximal MFM landed 5 cm before the brachiocephalic trunk and distally at the level of the aortoiliac bifurcation	The procedure with MFM involvement is shorter than conventional procedure with stent graft. There is much less total fluoroscopy time, less total contrast agent administered and a reduced risk of visceral embolization or branch dissection.
Sherif Sultan 2018 (Sultan et al. 2019)	investigated how the disease process can be modulated to equalize lumen pressure, enhance perfusion, and stabilize the aorta along its entire length using the kinetic elephant trunk (kET) technique that involving MFM in patients with chronic symptomatic aortic dissection (CSAD).	9	performed the kET on 9 patients with CSAD as a primary or secondary intervention, regardless of the chronicity of the dissection. examine the outcome. SMFM is deployed from the aortic sinus, covering the supra-aortic branches, distally into the distal aorta	kET is relatively safe in high-risk patients with low morbidity and mortality

Table 1. (Continued)

Author/Year	Study/objective	Patients with MFM	Methods used	Findings/Conclusion
Martinelli,2019 (Martinelli et al.)	To compare the results of open surgery and interventional endovascular strategies of visceral artery aneurysms in terms of technical success, therapy-associated complications and post- interventional follow-up in the elective and emergency.	2	Self-expandable multilayer stent was implanted in the common hepatic artery and in the SMA to preserve the PDA and the ileocolic artery, respectively. Stent and collateral pathways remained patent during follow-up	Two cases of using MFM shown promising results in terms of long lasting patenting in visceral aortic aneurysm and collateral pathways preservation.

Table 2. Clinical trials for the MFM and their current progress

Clinical Trial	Estimated timeline	Study model and subject recruited	Outcome of studies
Dragon Study Europe	Start Date: January 2016 Primary Completion Date: September 2018 Study Completion Date: September 2020	About 35 patients in up to 11 countries is expected to be enrolled and screened per the protocol-required inclusion and exclusion criteria, in order to achieve the target of 30 completed patients.	Ongoing (no outcome posted)
Evaluation of Safety and Efficacy of the Bifurcated Multilayer Flow Modulator (BMFM®). (STREAMLINER)	Start Date: April 2014 Primary Completion Date: June 2018 Study Completion Date: June 2022	This is an interventional (Clinical Trial) study. The actual enrollment is 42 participants	Ongoing (no outcome posted)
STRATO trial	Start Date: 01-03-2010 Completion Date: 01-04-2012 Primary Completion Date 01-04-2012	There are 23 cases of type II and III TAAAs treated with MFM with no aneurysm rupture. There is no migrations or fractures and no incidences of spinal cord ischemia, respiratory, renal, or peripheral complications.	A follow up report after 3 years show that endovascular repair with the MFM appears to be safe and effective while successfully maintaining branch vessel patency (Vaislic et al. 2016).

Overlapping Stents Treatment for Thoracic Aorta and Abdominal Aneurysm

Following the success of modulating flow patterns through MFM to reduce rupture, overlapping stents, which adopt a similar principle to MFM, have been designed and used to treat aortic aneurysms in China's Peking University Third Hospital. CT scans in the patients' follow-up visits showed stable thrombus in the aneurismal sac. The computational fluid dynamics (CFD) result showed no vortex formation in the aneurysm after implantation, as illustrated in Figure 9 (Zhang et al. 2014, Zhang et al. 2015). However, the long-term outcome remains unknown, since this method is only limited to a small cohort, and no published clinical results thus far have shown the success of overlapping stent technology. Zheng et al. performed the endovascular treatment of thoracoabdominal aortic aneurysm by the combination of a stent graft with overlapping bare-metal stents, and their results showed that the aneurysm had almost disappear with a flow preservation of four visceral arteries were achieved. It showed that overlapping bare metal stent can be a potential choice to treat TAAA in selected patients (Zeng, Huang, and He 2016). Another group from China has explored the efficacy and safety of multi-layer bare metal stents technique in the treatment of dissecting aneurysm involving visceral arteries (Dai et al. 2019). Their results from 16 cases showed that the treatment with multilayer bare-metal stents is safe with a higher patency rate of postoperative accumulated visceral arteries. A computational study also showed that deployment of three to four multilayer overlapping uncovered stents can help to create favorable hemodynamics environment to prevent rupture of fusiform aortic aneurysm while preserving patency of side branches (Yeow and Leo 2018). Another recent publication showed that overlapping stents can help to promote the growth of thrombus within the saccular aneurysm through changing the hemodynamic environment while leaving the branch unobstructed; however, more clinical evidence is required (Li et al. 2019). A clinical trial study, launched by Changhai Hospital in China to evaluate the safety and efficacy of multiple overlapping uncovered stents for endovascular pararenal aortic aneurysm repair, was started in May 2014 and is expected to be accomplished by October 2020. We expect to see more similar studies on overlapping stents to be launched to evaluate mid-term and long-term outcomes of using this approach.

Stent Graft with Perforations

Inspired by the MFM and overlapping stent strategy on smoothing the flow pattern, Leo's group proposed to build a stent graft design with perforations to treat aortic aneurysm (Ong et al. 2019, Ong, Ho, and Leo 2016). They have applied computational fluid dynamic (CFD) analysis to examine flow characteristics near the stented aortic arch in the simplified and patient-specific TAA models and compared that with *in-vitro* experimental results using particle image velocimetry (PIV) in a mock circulatory loop. The patency of side branches was maintained as demonstrated in *in-vitro* PIV results in Figure 3. The hemodynamics result was evaluated in terms of time-averaged wall shear stress (TAWSS) and endothelial cell action potential (ECAP) in Figures 4 and 5. Results showed that the stent graft with slit design can reduce the disturbed flow region considerably. Low TAWSS and elevated ECAP were observed on the aortic arch aneurysm after the placement, which implies the potential of thrombus formation in the aneurysm. On the other hand, the effects of the stent graft with full-slit design and half-slit design on shear stress did not vary significantly. Full-slit design has slits all over the entire circumference of SG, while half-slit design consisted of slits only on the top-half of the SG near the branching section. They decided to use the half-slit design for the experimental testing since it has a lower cost compared to the full-slits design. Their results indicated that the stent graft with slits not only shielded the aneurysm from rupture, but also resulted in a favorable environment for the thrombus that may contribute to the shrinkage of the aneurysm. The effect of the slit perforations on flow preservation to the supra-aortic branches was simulated and compared with the experimental results. The effectiveness of the stent graft with slits in maintaining flow patency at the branches was demonstrated by both simulation and experimental results, showing its potential for treating an aortic aneurysm involving proximity with branch vessels. This may ultimately benefit patients who are ineligible for currently available treatments, like branching and fenestrated stent grafts. The *in vivo* animal testing will be the next step in further developing this new concept design.

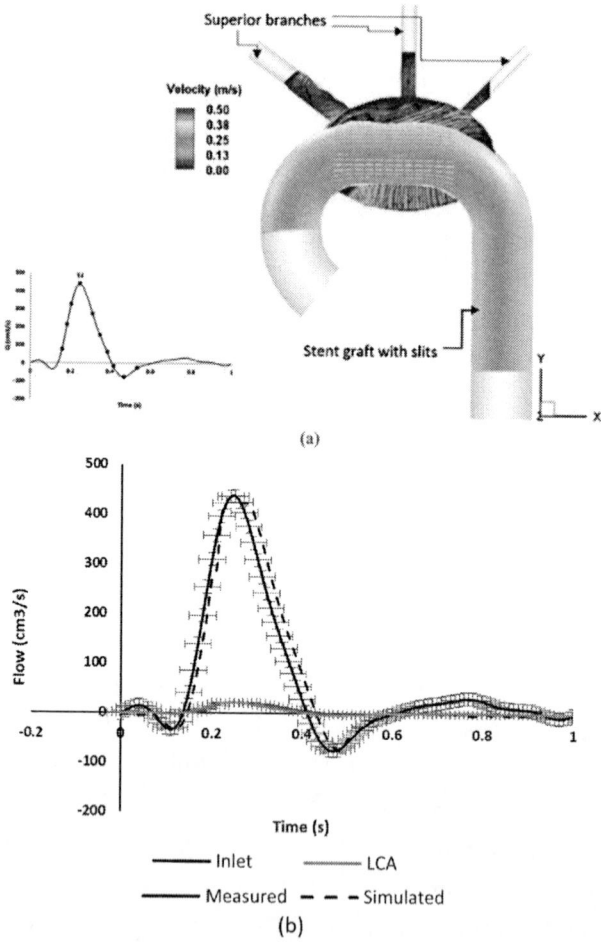

Figure 3. (a) The flow velocity field obtained from 3-D PIV in the mid-plane during peak systole (at T4). (b) Simulated and measured flow waveform at the inlet and left carotid common artery (LCA).

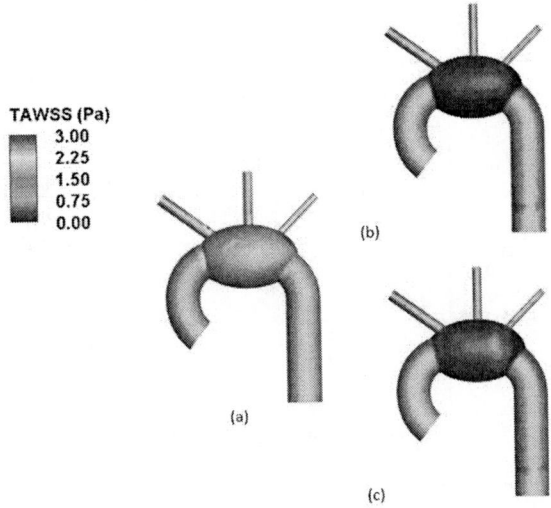

Figure 4. Contour maps of time-averaged wall shear stress (TAWSS) for (a) before treatment (b) half-slits and (c) full-slits.

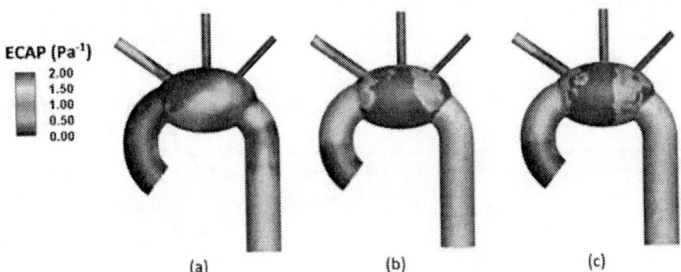

Figure 5. Contour maps of endothelial cell activation potential (ECAP) before and after the SG implantations (a) before treatment (b) half-slits (c) full-slits.

The flow pattern between the computational model and the PIV results in the patient-specific model was also compared. A middle plane is selected to present the differences of flow patterns. A good match between the flow patterns can be observed in Figure 6. Low-velocity (<0.13 m/s) region was found outside the aneurysm.

Table 3. Comparison chart for different surgical methods

Surgical method	Pros	Cons
Open surgery	Manage to prevent aneurysm rupture completely if surgery success	• Invasive method • Prolong hospitalization time
Hybrid repair	Avoid aortic cross-clamping Prolong ischemia time Suitable for patients refusing and unfit for open surgery	• Close monitoring of disease progress • Longer learning curve
Thoracic endovascular aneurysm repair (TEVAR)	Less invasive	• The safety and effectiveness are unsure
Branched and fenestrated stent graft	Preserve perfusion of aortic side branch	• Need custom made-devices • Complicated surgical procedures • Prone to proximal endoleak
Chimney repair	Prolong the sealing zone of aortic stent graft	• Type I endoleaks still occur • difficult to manufacture
Multilayer flow modulator	Reduce the risk of rupture by modulating the flow pattern	• Cannot immediately prevent rupture
Overlapping stents treatment	Reduce the risk of rupture by modulating the flow pattern	• Long term outcome unknown • Does not completely preserve the flow
Stent graft with slit perforations	Reduce the risk of rupture by modulating the flow pattern	• Only *in vitro* experiment demonstration, clinical trial not available

COMPARISON OF DIFFERENT TEVAR TREATMENT METHOD

In this section, we have compared the conventional treatment method with modern treatment methods, such as multilayer flow modulator and other methods, as shown in Table 3. We think even though the MFM inarguably is one of the potential candidates, it stills require more clinical trials to ensure the safety and effectiveness of the device.

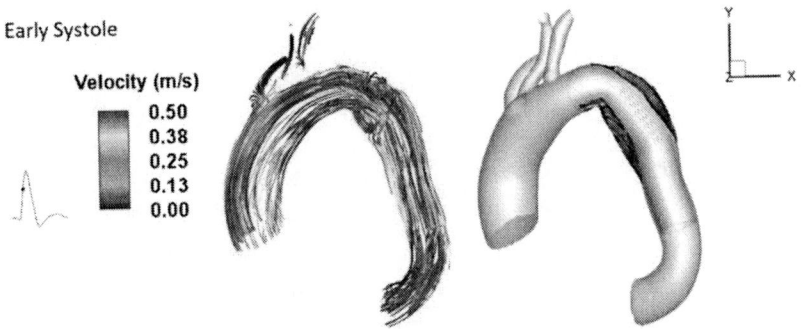

Figure 6. In-plane velocity pattern comparisons for the post treatment for the aneurysm at the early systole phase. Left: computational results Right: experimental results.

CONCLUSION

As observed in the evolution of any disruptive technology or innovation, there is always the need for large clinical or randomized trials to compare traditional repair with new endovascular interventions, so that the outcome of a new intervention is justifiable. The initiation of a large clinical trial for multilayer flow modular is a good step towards promising results. However, for the new therapy, even it was applied to a small number of cases of any these thoracic aortic pathologies, the results are still meaningful for surgeons to look at. As this chapter has shown, the results from technical study using computational fluid dynamics and operation in small number of patients are clear, as the new generation of proposed treatment working on the concept of smoothing flow pattern offers more flexibility to treat complex patient geometry with the potential of extending the landing zone of the stent graft. Endovascular treatment based on the flow pattern can be as reliable as well as durable in the management of aortic pathologies if it is used under IFU. Watchful follow-up is needed in all patients since the long-term outcome for these innovation devices has not been examined. A multicenter trial is recommended to verify the efficacy of a new generation of endovascular treatment. We also suggest a more comprehensive Instruction for use (IFU) and guidelines for these innovative techniques so that they can be used to treat multivariable aortic pathologies.

REFERENCES

Benjelloun, Amira, Michel Henry, Mustapha Taberkant, Abdelaziz Berrado, Rachid El Houati, and Abdelkader Semlali. 2016. "Multilayer flow modulator treatment of abdominal and thoracoabdominal aortic aneurysms with side branch coverage: outcomes from a prospective single-center Moroccan registry." *Journal of Endovascular Therapy* 23 (5):773-782. doi: 10.1177/1526602816657087.

Bishry, A. El, and H. Krebber. 2019. "Hybrid repair of aneurysms of aortic arch: is this the future treatment modality." *Heart, Lung and Circulation* 28:S69. doi: 10.1016/j.hlc.2019.02.015.

Browne, TF, D Hartley, S Purchas, M Rosenberg, G Van Schie, and M Lawrence-Brown. 1999. "A fenestrated covered suprarenal aortic stent." *European Journal of Vascular and Endovascular Surgery* 18 (5):445-449.

Calik, Eyupserhat, and Bilgehan Erkut. 2018. "Endovascular repair of a Stanford Type A dissection with the Cardiatis multilayer flow modulator." *Interactive CardioVascular and Thoracic Surgery* 28 (2):321-323. doi: 10.1093/icvts/ivy241.

Cardiatis. 2009. "*Outcomes*." http://www.cardiatis.com/?page_id=9.

Cavalcante, Rafael Noronha, Kenji Nishinari, Guilherme Yazbek, Mariana Krutman, Guilherme Bomfim, and Nelson Wolosker. 2015. "Severe visceral ischemia and death after multilayer stent deployment for the treatment of a thoracoabdominal aortic aneurysm." *Journal of Vascular Surgery* 62 (6):1632-1635.

Cheng, Davy, Janet Martin, Hani Shennib, Joel Dunning, Claudio Muneretto, Stephan Schueler, Ludwig Von Segesser, Paul Sergeant, and Marko Turina. 2010. "Endovascular aortic repair versus open surgical repair for descending thoracic aortic disease a systematic review and meta-analysis of comparative studies." *Journal of the American College of Cardiology* 55 (10):986-1001. doi: 10.1016/j.jacc.2009.11.047.

Costache, Victor S., Kak K. Yeung, Crina Solomon, Radu Popa, Tatiana Melnic, Mihai Sandu, Cristian Bucurenciu, Gabriela Candea, Adrian Santa, and Andreea Costache. 2018. "Aortic remodeling after total endovascular aortic repair with multilayer stents: computational fluid dynamics analysis of aortic remodeling over 3 years of follow-up." *Journal of Endovascular Therapy* 25 (6):760-764. doi: 10.1177/1526602818808049.

Czerny, Martin, Holger Eggebrecht, Gottfried Sodeck, Fabio Verzini, Piergiorgio Cao, Gabriele Maritati, Vicente Riambau, Friedhelm Beyersdorf, Bartosz Rylski, and Martin Funovics. 2012. "Mechanisms of symptomatic spinal cord ischemia after TEVAR: insights from the European Registry of Endovascular Aortic Repair Complications (EuREC)." *Journal of Endovascular Therapy* 19 (1):37-43.

Dai, Mingsheng, Tong Liu, Yudong Luo, Feng Zhou, Hailun Fan, Jiechang Zhu, Yiwei Zhang, Fanguo Hu, and Xiangchen Dai. 2019. "Treatment of aortic dissecting aneurysm involving visceral arteries with multi-layer bare stents." *Revista da Associação Médica Brasileira* 65 (2):216-221.

De Bakey, Michael E, and Denton A Cooley. 1953. "Successful resection of aneurysm of thoracic aorta and replacement by graft." *Journal of the American Medical Association* 152 (8):673-676.

Debing, E, D Aerden, S Gallala, F Vandenbroucke, and P Van den Brande. 2014. "Stenting complex aorta aneurysms with the Cardiatis multilayer flow modulator: first impressions." *European Journal of Vascular and Endovascular Surgery* 47 (6):604-608.

Diethrich, Edward B. 2014. "Present state of the multilayer flow modulator." in MEET, Arizona Heart Foundation: Phoenix, Arizona.

Eagleton, Matthew J. 2004. "*Thoracic Aortic Aneurysm.*" Accessed January 25th. https://vascular.org/patient-resources/vascular-conditions/thoracic-aortic-aneurysm.

Elkouri, Stephane, Peter Gloviczki, Michael A. McKusick, Jean M. Panneton, James Andrews, Thomas C. Bower, Audra A. Noel, William

S. Harmsen, Tanya L. Hoskin, and Kenneth Cherry. 2004. "Perioperative complications and early outcome after endovascular and open surgical repair of abdominal aortic aneurysms." *Journal of Vascular Surgery* 39 (3):497-505. doi: 10.1016/j.jvs.2003.10.018.

Greenberg, Roy K., Daniel Clair, Sunita Srivastava, Guru Bhandari, Adrian Turc, Jennifer Hampton, Matt Popa, Richard Green, and Kenneth Ouriel. 2003. "Should patients with challenging anatomy be offered endovascular aneurysm repair?" *Journal of Vascular Surgery* 38 (5):990-996. doi: http://dx.doi.org/10.1016/S0741-5214(03)00896-6.

Harvard, Publication Healthy. 2010. Shining a light on thoracic aortic disease - Harvard Health. *Harvard Health*.

Henry, Michel, Antonios Polydorou, Noureddine Frid, Patricia Gruffaz, Alain Cavet, Isabelle Henry, Michèle Hugel, Daniel A Rüfenacht, Luca Augsburger, and Matthieu De Beule. 2008. "Treatment of renal artery aneurysm with the multilayer stent." *Journal of Endovascular Therapy* 15 (2):231-236.

Hynes, Niamh, Sherif Sultan, Ala Elhelali, Edward B. Diethrich, Edel P. Kavanagh, Mohamed Sultan, Florian Stefanov, Patrick Delassus, and Liam Morris. 2016. "Systematic review and patient-level meta-analysis of the Streamliner multilayer flow modulator in the management of complex thoracoabdominal aortic pathology." *Journal of Endovascular Therapy* 23 (3):501-512. doi: 10.1177/1526602816636891.

Ibrahim, Walid, Konstantinos Spanos, Andreas Gussmann, Christoph A. Nienaber, Joerg Tessarek, Heinrich Walter, Jörg Thalwitzer, Sebastian E. Debus, Nikolaos Tsilimparis, and Tilo Kölbel. 2018. "Early and midterm outcome of Multilayer Flow Modulator stent for complex aortic aneurysm treatment in Germany." *Journal of Vascular Surgery* 68 (4):956-964. doi: 10.1016/j.jvs.2018.01.037.

Jonker, Frederik HW, Hence JM Verhagen, Peter H Lin, Robin H Heijmen, Santi Trimarchi, W Anthony Lee, Frans L Moll, Husam Atamneh, Vincenzo Rampoldi, and Bart E Muhs. 2011. "Open surgery versus endovascular repair of ruptured thoracic aortic aneurysms." *Journal of Vascular Surgery* 53 (5):1210-1216.

Kasemi, Holta, Mario Marino, Costantino Luca Di Angelo, Gian Franco Fadda, and Francesco Speziale. 2015. "Aortic arch and descending thoracic aortic saccular aneurysms treatment with fenestrated endograft and chimney technique for aortic branch rescue." *Annals of Vascular Surgery* 29 (1):126. e15-126. e19.

Kasipandian, V., and A. C. Pichel. 2012. "Complex endovascular aortic aneurysm repair." *Continuing Education in Anaesthesia, Critical Care & Pain* 12 (6):312-316. doi: 10.1093/bjaceaccp/mks035.

Kasprzak, P, K Gallis, B Cucuruz, K Pfister, M Janotta, and R Kopp. 2014. "Temporary aneurysm sac perfusion as an adjunct for prevention of spinal cord ischemia after branched endovascular repair of thoracoabdominal aneurysms." *Journal of Vascular Surgery* 60 (3).

Lazaris, Andreas M, Anastasios N Maheras, and Spyros N Vasdekis. 2012. "A multilayer stent in the aorta may not seal the aneurysm, thereby leading to rupture." *Journal of Vascular Surgery* 56 (3):829-831.

Li, Zhongyou, Lijuan Hu, Chong Chen, Zhenze Wang, Zhihong Zhou, and Yu Chen. 2019. "Hemodynamic performance of multilayer stents in the treatment of aneurysms with a branch attached." *Scientific Reports* 9 (1):10193. doi: 10.1038/s41598-019-46714-7.

Lindblad, B., A. Bin Jabr, J. Holst, and M. Malina. 2015. "Chimney grafts in aortic stent grafting: hazardous or useful technique? Systematic review of current data." *European Journal of Vascular and Endovascular Surgery* 50 (6):722-731. doi: http://dx.doi.org/10.1016/j.ejvs.2015.07.038.

Lioupis, Christos, and Cherrie Z Abraham. 2011. "Results and challenges for the endovascular repair of aortic arch aneurysms." *Perspectives in Vascular Surgery and Endovascular Therapy* 23 (3):202-213.

Lowe, C, A Worthington, F Serracino-Inglott, R Ashleigh, and C McCollum. 2016. "Multi-layer flow-modulating stents for thoraco-abdominal and peri-renal aneurysms: the UK pilot study." *European Journal of Vascular and Endovascular Surgery* 51 (2):225-231.

Martinelli, O., A. Giglio, L. Irace, A. Di Girolamo, B. Gossetti, and R. Gattuso. "Single-center experience in the treatment of visceral artery aneurysms." *Annals of Vascular Surgery*. doi: 10.1016/j.avsg.2019.01.010.

Melnic, Tatiana, Crina Solomon, Andreea Costache, Mihai Sandu, Cristian Bucurenciu, Gabriela Candea, Alexandru Slavu, and Victor Costache. 2018. "Total supra-aortic trunk coverage with new-generation multilayer stents for complex aortic diseases." *Journal of Vascular Surgery* 68 (5):e144. doi: 10.1016/j.jvs.2018.08.090.

Mitchell, R. Scott, Michael D. Dake, Charles P. Semba, Thomas J. Fogarty, Christopher K. Zarins, Robert P. Liddell, and D. Craig Miller. 1996. "Endovascular stent–graft repair of thoracic aortic aneurysms." *The Journal of Thoracic and Cardiovascular Surgery* 111 (5):1054-1062. doi: http://dx.doi.org/10.1016/S0022-5223(96)70382-3.

Morris, Liam, Florian Stefanov, Niamh Hynes, Edward B Diethrich, and Sherif Sultan. 2016. "An experimental evaluation of device/arterial wall compliance mismatch for four stent-graft devices and a multi-layer flow modulator device for the treatment of abdominal aortic aneurysms." *European Journal of Vascular and Endovascular Surgery* 51 (1):44-55.

Mozaffarian, Dariush, Emelia J. Benjamin, Alan S. Go, Donna K. Arnett, Michael J. Blaha, Mary Cushman, Sandeep R. Das, Sarah de Ferranti, Jean-Pierre Després, Heather J. Fullerton, Virginia J. Howard, Mark D. Huffman, Carmen R. Isasi, Monik C. Jiménez, Suzanne E. Judd, Brett M. Kissela, Judith H. Lichtman, Lynda D. Lisabeth, Simin Liu, Rachel H. Mackey, David J. Magid, Darren K. McGuire, Emile R. Mohler, Claudia S. Moy, Paul Muntner, Michael E. Mussolino, Khurram Nasir, Robert W. Neumar, Graham Nichol, Latha Palaniappan, Dilip K. Pandey, Mathew J. Reeves, Carlos J. Rodriguez, Wayne Rosamond, Paul D. Sorlie, Joel Stein, Amytis Towfighi, Tanya N. Turan, Salim S. Virani, Daniel Woo, Robert W. Yeh, and Melanie B. Turner. 2016. "Heart disease and stroke statistics—2016 update." *A Report From the American Heart Association* 133 (4):e38-e360. doi: 10.1161/cir.0000000000000350.

O'Callaghan, Adrian, Roy K. Greenberg, Matthew J. Eagleton, James Bena, and Tara Marie Mastracci. 2015. "Type Ia endoleaks after fenestrated and branched endografts may lead to component instability and increased aortic mortality." *Journal of Vascular Surgery* 61 (4):908-914. doi: http://dx.doi.org/10.1016/j.jvs.2014.10.085.

Ohrlander, Tomas, Björn Sonesson, Krasnodar Ivancev, Timothy Resch, Nuno Dias, and Martin Malina. 2008. "The chimney graft: A technique for preserving or rescuing aortic branch vessels in stent-graft sealing zones." *Journal of Endovascular Therapy* 15 (4):427-432. doi: 10.1583/07-2315.1.

Ong, Chi-Wei, Pei Ho, and Hwa-Liang Leo. 2016. "Effects of Microporous Stent Graft on the Descending Aortic Aneurysm: A Patient-Specific Computational Fluid Dynamics Study." *Artificial Organs* 40 (11):E230-E240. doi: 10.1111/aor.12802.

Ong, ChiWei, Fei Xiong, Foad Kabinejadian, Gideon Praveen Kumar, FangSen Cui, Gongfa Chen, Pei Ho, and HwaLiang Leo. 2019. "Hemodynamic analysis of a novel stent graft design with slit perforations in thoracic aortic aneurysm." *Journal of Biomechanics* 85:210-217. doi: https://doi.org/10.1016/j.jbiomech.2019.01.019.

Orozco-Sevilla, Vicente, Scott A. Weldon, and Joseph S. Coselli. 2018. "Hybrid thoracoabdominal aortic aneurysm repair: is the future here?" *Journal of Visualized Surgery* 4:61-61. doi: 10.21037/jovs.2018.02.14.

Oval, Cengiz, Aykut Sahin, Murat Eroglu, Sinan Balcm, Sadettin Dernek, and Mustafa Behcet Sevin. 2018. "Treatment of Aortic and Iliac Artery Aneurysms with Multilayer Flow Modulator: Single Centre Experiences." *International Journal of Vascular Medicine* 2018:9. doi: 10.1155/2018/7543817.

Ovalı, Cengiz, and Mustafa Behçet Sevin. 2018a. "The combined use of multilayer flow modulator stent and conventional stent grafts in complex thoracoabdominal aortic aneurysms and Type 3 dissections accompanying aneurysms." *Turkish Journal of Thoracic and Cardiovascular Surgery* 1 (1).

Ovalı, Cengiz, and Mustafa Behçet Sevin. 2018b. "A different approach to multilayer flow modulator implantation in aortic aneurysm." *Anatolian journal of cardiology* 19 (5):353-356. doi: 10.14744/AnatolJCardiol.2018.49274.

Parodi, Juan C, JC Palmaz, and HD Barone. 1991. "Transfemoral intraluminal graft implantation for abdominal aortic aneurysms." *Annals of Vascular Surgery* 5 (6):491-499.

Patel, Rakesh P., Athanasios Katsargyris, Eric L. G. Verhoeven, Donald J. Adam, and John A. Hardman. 2013. "Endovascular aortic aneurysm repair with chimney and snorkel grafts: indications, techniques and results." *CardioVascular and Interventional Radiology* 36 (6):1443-1451. doi: 10.1007/s00270-013-0648-5.

Pinto, Carolline, George Garas, Leanne Harling, Ara Darzi, Roberto Casula, and Thanos Athanasiou. 2017. "Is endovascular treatment with multilayer flow modulator stent insertion a safe alternative to open surgery for high-risk patients with thoracoabdominal aortic aneurysm?" *Annals of Medicine and Surgery* 15:1-8.

Quiñones-Baldrich, William J, Thomas F Panetta, Candace L Vescera, and Vikram S Kashyap. 1999. "Repair of type IV thoracoabdominal aneurysm with a combined endovascular and surgical approach." *Journal of Vascular Surgery* 30 (3):555-560.

Rikhtegar Nezami, Farhad, Lambros S. Athanasiou, Junedh M. Amrute, and Elazer R. Edelman. 2018. "Multilayer flow modulator enhances vital organ perfusion in patients with type B aortic dissection." *American Journal of Physiology-Heart and Circulatory Physiology* 315 (5):H1182-H1193. doi: 10.1152/ajpheart.00199.2018.

Rolph, Rachel, James Duffy, Bijan Modarai, Rachel E Clough, Peter Taylor, and Matthew Waltham. 2013. "Stent graft types for endovascular repair of thoracic aortic aneurysms." *The Cochrane Library*.

Schafigh, Myriam Johanna, Zaki Kohistani, Wolfgang Schiller, and Chris Probst. 2018. "Retrograde Stanford type A dissection caused by a multilayer stent graft in a patient with chronic type B dissection." *Interactive CardioVascular and Thoracic Surgery* 28 (4):655-656. doi: 10.1093/icvts/ivy313.

Scurr, James R. H., and Richard G. McWilliams. 2007. "Fenestrated aortic stent grafts." *Seminars in Interventional Radiology* 24 (2):211-220. doi: 10.1055/s-2007-980049.

Sherif Sultan, MCh, Edel P Kavanagh, Victor Costache, Mohamed Sultan, Edward Diethrich, Fionnuala Jordan, and Niamh Hynes. 2017. "Streamliner multilayer flow modulator for thoracoabdominal aortic pathologies: recommendations for revision of indications and contraindications for use." *Vascular Disease Management* 14 (4):E90-E99.

Spinella, Giovanni, Alice Finotello, Elena Faggiano, Bianca Pane, Michele Conti, Valerio Gazzola, Ferdinando Auricchio, and Domenico Palombo. 2018. "Midterm Follow-up Geometrical Analysis of Thoracoabdominal Aortic Aneurysms Treated with Multilayer Flow Modulator." *Annals of Vascular Surgery* 53:97-104.e2. doi: 10.1016/j.avsg.2018.04.034.

Stefanov, Florian, Liam Morris, Ala Elhelali, Edel P Kavanagh, Violet Lundon, Niamh Hynes, and Sherif Sultan. 2016. "Insights from complex aortic surgery with a Streamliner device for aortic arch repair (STAR)." *The Journal of Thoracic and Cardiovascular Surgery* 152 (5):1309-1318. e5.

Sultan, Sherif, and Niamh Hynes. 2013. "One-year results of the multilayer flow modulator stent in the management of thoracoabdominal aortic aneurysms." *Journal of Vascular Surgery* 57 (5):19S. doi: 10.1016/j.jvs.2013.02.067.

Sultan, Sherif, Niamh Hynes, Edel P Kavanagh, and Edward B Diethrich. 2014. "How does the multilayer flow modulator work? The science behind the technical innovation." *Journal of Endovascular Therapy* 21 (6):814-821.

Sultan, Sherif, Niamh Hynes, and Mohamed Sultan. 2014. "When not to implant the multilayer flow modulator: lessons learned from application outside the indications for use in patients with thoracoabdominal pathologies." *Journal of Endovascular Therapy* 21 (1):96-112.

Sultan, Sherif, Edel P Kavanagh, Michel Bonneau, Chantal Kang, Antoine Alves, and Niamh Hynes. 2014. "Assessment of biocompatibility of the multilayer flow modulator with differing thread designs." *Journal of Vascular Medicine & Surgery*.

Sultan, Sherif, Edel P Kavanagh, Michel Bonneau, Chantal Kang, Antoine Alves, and Niamh M Hynes. 2016. "Kinetics of endothelialization of the multilayer flow modulator and single-layer arterial stents." *Vascular* 24 (1):78-87.

Sultan, Sherif, Edel P. Kavanagh, Dave Veerasingam, Victor Costache, Ala Elhelali, Brian Fitzgibbon, Edward Diethrich, and Niamh Hynes. 2019. "Kinetic Elephant Trunk Technique: Early Results in Chronic Symptomatic Aortic Dissection Management." *Annals of Vascular Surgery* 57:244-252. doi: 10.1016/j.avsg.2018.08.083.

Swan, Henry, clarence Maaske, marvin Johnson, and robert Grover. 1950. "Arterial homografts: II. Resection of thoracic aortic aneurysm using a stored human arterial transplant." *AMA Archives of Surgery* 61 (4):732-737.

Swerdlow, Nicholas J, Winona W Wu, and Marc L Schermerhorn. 2019. "Open and endovascular management of aortic aneurysms." *Circulation Research* 124 (4):647-661.

Tirziu, Daniela, Rodney White, William Gray, Cody Pietras, Mohammed Imran Ghare, and Alexandra Lansky. 2018. "Endovascular repair of penetrating atherosclerotic ulcers with the cardiatis multilayer flow modulator implant as an alternative to covered endografts to preserve branch vessel patency." *Journal of the American College of Cardiology* 72 (13 Supplement):B38.

Tshomba, Yamume, Germano Melissano, Davide Logaldo, Enrico Rinaldi, Luca Bertoglio, Efrem Civilini, Daniele Psacharopulo, and Roberto Chiesa. 2012. "Clinical outcomes of hybrid repair for thoracoabdominal aortic aneurysms." *Annals of Cardiothoracic Surgery* 1 (3):293-303.

Ucci, Alessandro, Ruggiero Curci, Matteo Azzarone, Claudio Bianchini Massoni, Antonio Bozzani, Carla Marcato, Enrico Maria Marone, Paolo Perini, Tiziano Tecchio, Antonio Freyrie, and Angelo Argenteri. 2018. "Early and mid-term results in the endovascular treatment of popliteal aneurysms with the multilayer flow modulator." *Vascular* 26 (5):556-563. doi: 10.1177/1708538118771258.

Vaislic, Claude D., Jean Noël Fabiani, Sidney Chocron, Jacques Robin, Victor S. Costache, Jean-Pierre Villemot, Jean Marc Alsac, Pascal N. Leprince, Thierry Unterseeh, Eric Portocarrero, Yves Glock, and Hervé Rousseau. 2016. "Three-Year Outcomes with the Multilayer Flow

Modulator for Repair of Thoracoabdominal Aneurysms: A Follow-up Report from the STRATO Trial." *Journal of Endovascular Therapy* 23 (5):762-772. doi: 10.1177/1526602816653095.

Yeow, Siang Lin, and Hwa Liang Leo. 2018. "Is multiple overlapping uncovered stents technique suitable for aortic aneurysm repair?" *Artificial Organs* 42 (2):174-183. doi: 10.1111/aor.12993.

Yoshitake, Akihiro, Yasunori Iida, Masataka Yamazaki, Kanako Hayashi, Yu Inaba, and Hideyuki Shimizu. 2019. "Midterm results of 2-stage hybrid arch repair for extensive aortic arch aneurysms." *Annals of Vascular Surgery* 56:97-102. doi: https://doi.org/10.1016/j.avsg.2018.07.063.

Zeng, Wei, Shan Huang, and Chunshui He. 2016. "Endovascular Treatment of Thoracoabdominal Aorta Aneurysm by the Combination of a Stent Graft with Multiple Overlapping Bare Stents." *Annals of Vascular Surgery* 36:289.e1-289.e4. doi: https://doi.org/10.1016/j.avsg.2016.02.029.

Zhang, Peng, Xiao Liu, Anqiang Sun, Yubo Fan, and Xiaoyan Deng. 2015. "Hemodynamic insight into overlapping bare-metal stents strategy in the treatment of aortic aneurysm." *J Biomech* 48 (10):2041-2046.

Zhang, Peng, Anqiang Sun, Fan Zhan, Jingyuan Luan, and Xiaoyan Deng. 2014. "Hemodynamic study of overlapping bare-metal stents intervention to aortic aneurysm." *J Biomech* 47 (14):3524-3530.

BIOGRAPHICAL SKETCH

Leo Hwa Liang

Affiliation: National University of Singapore

Education: PhD in Bioengineering, Georgia Institute of Technology, Atlanta, Georgia

Research and Professional Experience:

My research focus is the integration of biofluid mechanics with the development of medical devices. One of the several applications centers on the development of implantable devices to be used in areas of cardiovascular circulation and interventional cardiology. My research interests also include the fluid mechanical assessment of cardiovascular devices and therapeutics interventions, and the study of the hemodynamics origin of various cardiovascular diseases. At present, I am designing and developing novel heart valve prosthesis and vascular stents for percutaneous implantation. My other research interests and expertise center on the design and development of bioreactors and novel in vitro system for drug screening and toxicological testing. These works involve the use of computational fluid dynamics simulations and experimental setups for the characterization and optimization of the cell culturing systems.

Professional Appointments: Associate Professor at National University of Singapore

Honors:

2014/2015	NUS Faculty of Engineering Teaching Award (Commendation List)
Dec 2013	NUS, Faculty of Engineering on Innovative Teaching Award 2013 (Silver)
Aug 2009	Asia Pacific Traveling Fellowship, International Federation for Medical and Biological Engineering
June 2003 - Dec 2004	International Fellowship, Agency for Science, Technology and Research (ASTAR)
Dec 2002	International Congress on Biology and Medical Engineering (ICBME) Young Investigator Award Winner in Category: Biomechanics/BioMEMS
Aug 1999 - May 2005	Georgia Institute of Technology Graduate Research Assistantship
Apr 1996 - June 1999	Nanyang Technological University Graduate Research Scholarship

Publications from the Last 3 Years:

1. H. Wiputra, C. K. Chen, E. Talbi, G. L. Lim, S. Soomar, A. Biswas, C. Mattar, D. Bark, H. L. Leo, and C. H. Yap, 'Human Fetal Hearts with Tetralogy of Fallot have Altered Fluid Dynamics and Forces,' submitted to *American Journal of Physiology – Heart,* June 2018.
2. Y. L. Shao, H. L. Leo, K. J. Chua, 'Studying of the thermal performance of a hybrid cryo RFA treatment of a solid tumor,' *International Journal of Heat and Mass Transfer* 122, 410-420, 2018.
3. C. W. Ong, C. H. Yap, F. Kabinejadian, Y. N. Nguyen, F. Cui, K. J. Chua, P. Ho and H. L. Leo, 'Association of Hemodynamic Behavior in the Thoracic Aortic Aneurysm to the Intraluminal Thrombus Prediction: A Two-Way Fluid Structure Coupling Investigation,' *International Journal of Applied Mechanics* 10(4):01 May 2018, Corresponding author.
4. B. Namgung, Y. C. Ng, H. L. Leo, J. M. Rifkind, S. Kim, 'Near-Wall Migration Dynamics of Erythrocytes in Vivo: Effects of Cell Deformability and Arteriolar Bifurcation,' *Frontiers In Physiology* 8:10 pages Number ARTN 963 29 Nov 2017.
5. Y. N. Nguyen, Ismail M, Kabinejadian, C. W. Ong, E. L. W. Tay, H. L. Leo, 'Experimental Study of Right Ventricular Hemodynamics After Tricuspid Valve Replacement Therapies to Treat Tricuspid Regurgitation,' *Cardiovascular Engineering and Technology* 8(4):401-418 01 Dec 2017, Corresponding author.
6. Y. L. Shao, B. Arjun, H. L. Leo, K. J. A. Chua, 'A Computational Theoretical Model For Radiofrequency Ablation Of Tumor With Complex Vascularization,' *Computers in Biology and Medicine* 89:282-292 01 Oct 2017.
7. Justin K. S. Tan, H. L. Leo and S. Kim, 'Continuous Separation of White Blood Cells from Whole Blood Using Viscoelastic Effects,' *IEEE Transactions On Biomedical Circuits And Systems*, Vol. X, No. 1, November 2017.

8. C. H. Yap, H. Wiputra, G. L. ing LIM; K. C. Chua, N. Raju, S. M. Soomar, A. Biswas, C. N. Z. Mattar, H. L. Leo, 'Peristaltic-Like Motion of the Human Fetal Right Ventricle and its Effects on Fluid Dynamics and Energy Dynamics, *Annals Of Biomedical Engineering* 45(10):2335-2347 (13 pages) 01 Oct 2017.
9. M. Ismail, F. Kabinejadian, Y. N. Nguyen, L. W. Tay, H. L. Leo, 'Design and Development of Novel Transcatheter Bi-Caval Valves in the Interventional Treatment of Tricuspid Regurgitation,' *Artificial Organs*, September 11, 2017, Corresponding author.
10. Y. N. Nguyen, M. Ismail, F. Kabinejadian, L. W. Tay and H. L. Leo, 'Experimental Study of Right Ventricular Hemodynamics After Tricuspid Valve Replacement Therapies to Treat Tricuspid Regurgitation,' accepted, *Cardiovascular Engineering and Technology,* 2017 Dec;8(4):401-418. 2017, Corresponding author.
11. S. L. Yeow; S. Y. Benjamin Chua, H. L. Leo, 'Is multiple overlapping uncovered stents technique suitable for aortic aneurysm repair?,' *Artificial Organs*, September 11, 2017. Corresponding author.

Ong Chi Wei

Affiliation: National University of Singapore

Education: PhD in Biomedical Engineering (ongoing)

Research and Professional Experience:

Dr. Ong research interests are in computational and experimental biofluid mechanics. Currently he is working as research fellow in NUS on modelling fetal mechanics. He has over seven years of research expertise in the computational study of the development of various medical devices, such as stents design and left ventricular assist devices. His Ph.D. focuses on the hemodynamic interrogations for the novel preferential covered stent design implanted in aortic aneurysms from a computational and experimental perspective. Other projects he has collaborated with clinicians in various hospital in Singapore in studying the impact of stent design in the carotid artery and developing the fluid-structure interaction framework to model the interaction between the synovial fluid and wrist bone. He worked in a deep tech start-up company as apprentice to help segment and simulate the flow in cerebral aneurysm through machine learning and computational fluid dynamics before joining NUS as research fellow.

Professional Appointments: Research Fellow in National University of Singapore

Honors:
2015~2019 AUN/SEED-Net Graduate Scholarship in Singapore

Publications from the Last 3 Years:

1. Chi Wei Ong, Fei Xiong, Foad Kabinejadian, Gideon Praveen Kumar, FangSen Cui, Gongfa Chen, Pei Ho, Hwa Liang Leo. (2019). Hemodynamic Analysis of a Novel Stent Graft Design with Slit Perforations in Thoracic Aortic Aneurysm. *Journal of Biomechanics*
2. Chi Wei Ong, Foad Kabinejadian, Fei Xiong, Yoke Rung Wong, Milan Toma, Yen Ngoc Nguyen, FangSen Cui, Pei Ho, Hwa Liang Leo. (2019) Pulsatile Flow Investigation in Development of Thoracic Aortic Aneurysm: An *In-Vitro* Validated Fluid Structure Interaction Analysis. *Journal of Applied Fluid Mechanics*
3. Chi Wei Ong, Choon Hwai Yap, Foad Kabinejadian, Yen Ngoc Nguyen, Fangsen Cui, Kian Jon Chua, Pei Ho, and Hwa Liang Leo (2018). Association of hemodynamic behavior in the thoracic aortic aneurysm to the intraluminal thrombus prediction: A two-way fluid structure coupling investigation. *International Journal of Applied Mechanics*, 1850035.

4. Chi Wei Ong, Pei Ho., & Hwa Liang Leo (2016). Effects of Microporous Stent Graft on the Descending Aortic Aneurysm: A Patient-Specific Computational Fluid Dynamics Study. *Artificial Organs*, 40(11).
5. Tseng, Fan Shuen, Tse Kiat Soong, Nicholas Syn, Chi Wei Ong, Leo Hwa Liang, and Andrew MTL Choong. "Computational fluid dynamics in complex aortic surgery: applications, prospects and challenges." *Journal of Surgical Simulation* 4 (2017): 1-4.
6. Yeong Xue Lun, Ko Teck Ee Reyor, Chi Wei Ong, Leo Hwa Liang, Andrew M. T. L. Choong (2017). The importance of 3D printing in vascular surgical simulation and training. *Journal of Surgical Simulation,* 4, 23-28.
7. Nguyen, Yen Ngoc, Munirah Ismail, Foad Kabinejadian, Chi Wei Ong, Edgar Lik Wui Tay, and Hwa Liang Leo. "Experimental Study of Right Ventricular Hemodynamics After Tricuspid Valve Replacement Therapies to Treat Tricuspid Regurgitation." *Cardiovascular engineering and technology* (2017): 1-18.

Foad Kabinejadian

Affiliation: Tulane University

Education: PhD in Mechanical Engineering, Nanyang Technological University, Singapore

Research and Professional Experience:

Dr. Kabinejadian has more than ten years of experience in biomedical research, contributing to and leading projects on design, test, and development of novel medical devices. The primary scope of his research includes experimental, analytical, and computational cardiovascular and biofluid mechanics. He has extensive research experience on abdominal aortic aneurysm, intracranial carotid aneurysm, and design of aortic valves, mitral valves, and flow modulator covered stents. More recently, he has started research on treatment of hepatocellular carcinoma utilizing acoustic droplet vaporization by focused ultrasound in the tumor to induce targeted ischemia.

Professional Appointments: Postdoctoral Research Fellow at Tulane University

Honors:

- First Prize Winner, "MIT HackMed @ SG," the first MIT Hacking Medicine healthcare hackathon in Singapore, 7/2015
- Thematic Prize Winner for best addressing the "Aging-in-Place" Challenge Statement, "MIT HackMed @ SG," 7/2015
- Full Graduate Research Scholarship Award, Granted by Nanyang Technological University, Singapore, 1/2007 to 1/2011

Publications from the Last 3 Years:

1. Ong, C. W., F. Kabinejadian, F. Xiong, Y. R. Wong, M. Toma, Y. N. Nguyen, K. J. Chua, F. S. Cui, P. Ho, and H. L. Leo. "Pulsatile Flow Investigation in Development of Thoracic Aortic Aneurysm: An In-Vitro Validated Fluid Structure Interaction Analysis," *Journal of Applied Fluid Mechanics*, 2019 (Accepted).
2. Ong, C. W., F. Xiong, F. Kabinejadian, G. P. Kumar, F. S. Cui, G. Chen, P. Ho, and H. L. Leo. "Hemodynamic Analysis of a Novel Stent Graft Design with Slit Perforations in Thoracic Aortic Aneurysm," *Journal of Biomechanics* 85, pp. 120–127, 2019.
3. Su, B., X. Wang, F. Kabinejadian, C. Chin, T. T. Le, and J. M. Zhang. "Effects of left atrium on intraventricular flow in numerical simulations," *Computers in Biology and Medicine*, 2019 (Accepted).
4. Ismail, M., F. Kabinejadian, Y. N. Nguyen, and H. L. Leo. "Design and Development of Novel Transcatheter Bi-Caval Valves in the

Interventional Treatment of Tricuspid Regurgitation," *Artificial Organs* 42(2), pp. E13–E28, 2018.

5. Nguyen, Y. N., M. Ismail, F. Kabinejadian, E. L. Tay, and H. L. Leo. "Post-Operative Ventricular Flow Dynamics following Atrioventricular Valve Surgical and Device Therapies: A Review," *Medical Engineering & Physics* 54, pp. 1-13, 2018.

6. Ong, C. W., C. H. Yap, F. Kabinejadian, Y. N. Nguyen, F. Cui, K. J. Chua, P. Ho, and H. L. Leo. "Association of Hemodynamic Behavior in the Thoracic Aortic Aneurysm to the Intraluminal Thrombus Prediction: A Two-Way Fluid Structure Coupling Investigation," *International Journal of Applied Mechanics* 10(4), 2018.

7. Harmon, J. S., F. Kabinejadian, R. Seda, M. L. Fabiilli, S. P. Kuruvilla, J. M. Greve, B. J. Fowlkes, J. L. Bull. "Gas Embolization in a Rodent Model of Hepatocellular Carcinoma Using Acoustic Droplet Vaporization," *40th Annual International Conference of the IEEE Engineering in Medicine and Biology Society (EMBC)*, Honolulu, HI, 2018, pp. 6048-6051.

8. Kabinejadian, F., B. Su, D. N. Ghista, M. Ismail, S. Kim, and H. L. Leo. "Sequential venous anastomosis design to enhance patency of arterio-venous grafts for hemodialysis," *Computer Methods in Biomechanics and Biomedical Engineering* 20(1), pp. 85-93, 2017.

9. Ruiz-Soler, F. Kabinejadian, and A. Keshmiri. "Optimization of a Novel Spiral-Inducing Bypass Graft Using Computational Fluid Dynamics," *Scientific Reports,* 7:1865, 2017.

10. Ismail, M., F. Kabinejadian, Y. N. Nguyen, E. L. Tay, S. Kim, and H. L. Leo. "Hemodynamic assessment of extra-cardiac tricuspid valves using particle image velocimetry," *Medical Engineering and Physics* 50, pp. 1-11, 2017.

11. Nguyen, Y. N., M. Ismail, F. Kabinejadian, C. W. Ong, E. L. W. Tay, and H. L. Leo. "Investigating Right Ventricular Hemodynamics following Tricuspid Valve Replacement Therapies to treat Functional Tricuspid Regurgitation," *Cardiovascular Engineering and Technology* 8(4), pp. 401-418, 2017.

12. Kabinejadian, F., M. Kaabi Nezhadian, F. Cui, P. Ho, and H. L. Leo. "Covered Stent Membrane Design for Treatment of Atherosclerotic Disease at Carotid Artery Bifurcation and Prevention of Thromboembolic Stroke: An In Vitro Experimental Study," *Artificial Organs* 40(2), pp. 159-168, 2016.
13. Kabinejadian, F., M. McElroy, A. Ruiz-Soler, H. L. Leo, M. Slevin, L. Badimon, and A. Keshmiri. "Numerical Assessment of Novel Helical/Spiral Grafts with Improved Hemodynamics for Distal Graft Anastomoses," *PLOS ONE* 11(11): e0165892, 2016.
14. Kumar, G. P., F. Kabinejadian, J. Liu, P. Ho, H. L. Leo, F. Cui. "Simulated Bench Testing to Evaluate the Mechanical Performance of New Carotid Stents," *Artificial Organs*, 2016.
15. Ismail, M., G. P. Kumar, F. Kabinejadian, Y. N. Nguyen, F. Cui, E. L. W. Tay, and H. L. Leo. "An Experimental and Computational Study on the Effect of Caval Valved Stent Oversizing," *Cardiovascular Engineering and Technology* 7(3), pp. 254-269, 2016.

Ala Elhelali

Affiliation: John Hopkin University

Education: PhD in Biomedical Engineering, Galway Mayo Institute of Technology, Ireland

Research and Professional Experience:

Dr. Elhelali is a postdoctoral research fellow at Johns Hopkins University in the Department of Plastic and Reconstructive Surgery. She received her doctorate in Biomedical Engineering from Galway Mayo Institute of Technology. Her doctoral work focused on the experimental investigation of complex patient specific aortic arch aneurysm treated with the Cardiatis multilayer flow modulator. She was awarded the Health

Research Board (HRB) Ireland Cochrane Fellowship in 2016 and subsequently has worked on two systematic reviews focusing on surgical interventions for thoracic aortic arch aneurysms and dissections. In her current role at Johns Hopkins University, Department of Plastic and Reconstructive Surgery, she is involved in coordinating and performing clinical research aimed at developing therapies for peripheral nerve injuries.

Professional Appointments: Postdoctoral Research Fellow at John Hopkins University

Honors:

2016-2018 Health Research Board (HRB) Ireland Cochrane Fellow

Publications from the Last 3 Years:

1. Klifto KM, Elhelali A, Gurno CF, Seal SM, Asif M, Hultman CS. Acute surgical vs non-surgical management for ocular and peri-ocular burns: a systematic review and meta-analysis. *Burns & trauma*. 2019 Dec 1;7(1):25.
2. Sultan S, Kavanagh EP, Veerasingam D, Costache V, Elhelali A, Fitzgibbon B, Diethrich E, Hynes N. Kinetic Elephant Trunk Technique: Early Results in Chronic Symptomatic Aortic Dissection Management. *Annals of vascular surgery*. 2019 May 1;57:244-52.
3. Klifto KM, Major MR, Barone AA, Payne RM, Elhelali A, Seal SM, Cooney CM, Manahan MA, Rosson GD. Perioperative systemic nonsteroidal anti-inflammatory drugs (NSAIDs) in women undergoing breast surgery. *Cochrane Database of Systematic Reviews*. 2019(3).
4. Kavanagh EP, Jordan F, Hynes N, Elhelali A, Devane D, Veerasingam D, Sultan S. Hybrid repair versus conventional open repair for aortic arch dissection. *Cochrane Database of Systematic Reviews*. 2018(1).

5. Elhelali A, Hynes N, Devane D, Sultan S, Kavanagh EP, Morris L, Veerasingam D, Jordan F. Hybrid repair versus conventional open repair for thoracic aortic arch aneurysms. *Cochrane Database of Systematic Reviews*. 2018(1).
6. Sultan S, Kavanagh EP, Stefanov F, Sultan M, Elhelali A, Costache V, Diethrich E, Hynes N, Petrov I, Grozdinski L, Moosdorf R. Endovascular management of chronic symptomatic aortic dissection with the Streamliner Multilayer Flow Modulator: twelve-month outcomes from the global registry. *Journal of vascular surgery*. 2017 Apr 1;65(4):940-50.
7. Stefanov F, Sultan S, Morris L, Elhelali A, Kavanagh EP, Lundon V, Sultan M, Hynes N. Computational fluid analysis of symptomatic chronic type B aortic dissections managed with the Streamliner Multilayer Flow Modulator. *Journal of vascular surgery*. 2017 Apr 1;65(4):951-63.
8. Sultan S, Costache V, Kavanagh EP, ElHelali A, Hynes N. Twelve-Month Outcome From the MFM Global Registry on Endovascular Management of Chronic Symptomatic Aortic Dissection With the Streamliner Multilayer Flow Modulator. *Journal of Vascular Surgery*. 2017 Mar 1;65(3):e6.

In: Aortic Aneurysms
Editor: Amer Harky

ISBN: 978-1-53617-677-3
© 2020 Nova Science Publishers, Inc.

Chapter 3

ABDOMINAL AORTIC ANEURYSMS: MORPHOLOGY, RISK FACTORS, MANAGEMENT AND IMAGE-BASED MODELING STRATEGIES

Golnaz Jalalahmadi[1], María Helguera[1,2] and Cristian A. Linte[1,3,]*

[1]Chester F. Carlson Center for Imaging Science,
Rochester Institute of Technology, Rochester, NY, US
[2]Instituto Tecnológico José Mario Molina Pasquel y Henríquez – Unidad Lagos de Moreno, Jalisco, México
[3]Biomedical Engineering Department,
Rochester Institute of Technology, Rochester, NY, US

ABSTRACT

Abdominal aortic aneurysms (AAAs) are degenerative expansions of the infra-renal region of aorta. It has been suggested that various types of

---

* Corresponding Author's Email: gj2276@rit.edu & calbme@rit.edu.

parameters contribute to the weakening of the vessel wall and growth of the AAA, eventually leading to fatal AAA rupture. In this chapter, we review the AAA morphology and the three main categories of parameters that influence AAA behavior, including geometrical indices, biomechanical parameters, and lifestyle and health history. We also review different strategies for monitoring and managing AAA progression, and available treatment options.

Keywords: abdominal aortic aneurysm, geometrical indices, biomechanical parameters, life-style and health factors, morphology, treatment, imaging

INTRODUCTION

Abdominal aortic aneurysms (AAAs) are characterized by dilations of the abdominal aorta, typically within the infra-renal region of the vessel, that cause an expansion of at least 1.5 times the normal vessel diameter (Polzer and Gasser 2015; Ramadan, Al-Omran, and Verma 2017; Bogunovic et al. 2019; Tang et al. 2019). Figure 1b shows a three-dimensional CT angiogram of an infra-renal AAA for a specific patient in comparison with a normal AAA (Figure 1a).

AAAs occur in up to 2% of women and up to 8% of men 65 years old and older (Villard and Hultgren 2018; Tang et al. 2019; Sprynger et al. 2019). However, the mortality rate has shown an increase among younger patients (Vu et al. 2014). AAAs are typically asymptomatic, and, if undetected and left untreated, they pose a high risk of rupture, leading to a mortality rate of about 85-90% (Bogunovic et al. 2019; de Figueiredo et al. 2019; Kazimierczak et al. 2019). Moreover, while timely surgical repair is the preferred treatment approach, the risk of mortality for patients undergoing AAA repair surgery could be as high as 80% within 30 days of the procedure (Niestrawska et al. 2016; Leemans et al. 2017; Wilson et al. 2017).

In 2009, as a result of the high risk of rupture of AAAs, the Society for Vascular Surgery (SVS) practice guidelines expressed the critical need to further investigate the factors associated with the risk of AAA rupture, along with potential treatment methods (Chaikof et al. 2009; Zeinali-Davarani, Raguin, and Vorp 2011; Tang et al. 2014).

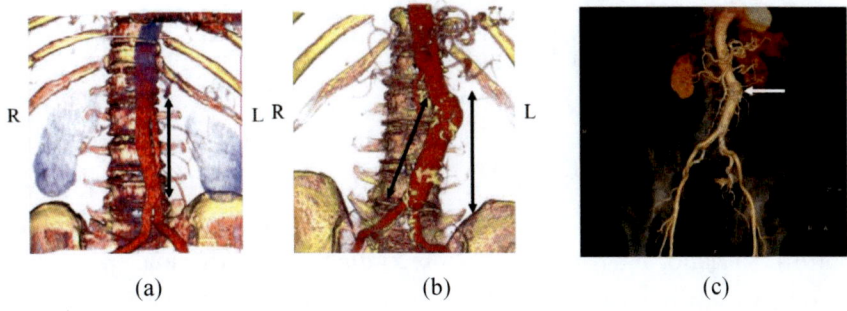

(a) (b) (c)

Figure 1. Volume rendered 3D CT generated from a patient-specific dataset using 3D Slicer, showing in (a) a normal straight abdominal aorta, in (b) an aneurysm evidenced by the inclined and bulged abdominal aorta, and (c) 3D rendition of infra-renal abdominal aortic aneurysm (indicated with white arrow).

This chapter is intended to serve as a comprehensive review of AAA physiology, behavior, and clinical management from an engineering perspective. A detailed discussion on morphological phenomena that initiate the progression of abdominal aortic aneurysm (AAA) will be presented, followed by an overview of different geometrical, biomechanical, and morphological parameters that affect AAA. Lastly, an overview of various modeling techniques that have evolved to date in response to different imaging-based screening and follow-up methods, as well as different strategies for clinical management and treatment of AAA will also be visited.

It has been hypothesized that the main reason attributed to the development of AAAs was the growing weakness of the aortic wall due to the metabolic activity of the metalloproteinase matrix at the aneurysm site (Fillinger et al. 2003; Tang et al. 2014; Farotto et al. 2018). This remodeling process leads to progressive degradation of elastin and collagen that make up the structural load bearing components of the aortic wall, resulting in a reduced compliance of the aortic wall tissue. The reduction in distensibility changes the strength distribution of the aortic wall and its stress bearing capacity, hence compromising its ability to tolerate and absorb large deformations caused by high pressure and inherent internal stresses. The ultimate result is often referred to "buckling" of the vessel wall, producing an aneurysm that essentially poses a high risk of rupture, lethal to patients (Heng et al. 2008; Bihari et al. 2013; Stevens et al. 2017; Wittek et al. 2018; Tang et al. 2019; Bogunovic et al. 2019).

Traditionally, the maximal transverse diameter (D_{max}) of the AAA sac has been considered as the main feature to monitor AAA progression as part of the clinical management of the condition, as well as assessing the need for surgical repair (Martufi et al. 2009; Tang et al. 2014; Shum et al. 2011; Martufi, Satriano, and Moore 2015). According to this criterion, D_{max} values of up to 5.5 cm suggest minimal risk, while a D_{max} higher than 5.5 cm is an indicator of high rupture risk. More specifically, a D_{max} of 5.5 cm in men or 4.9 - 5.0 cm in women, accompanied by an expansion rate of 1.0 cm/year, are considered high risk factor indicators and a biomarker threshold to justify the cost of elective repair (Martufi et al. 2009; Koncar et al. 2012; Engelbergera et al. 2017; Wu et al. 2019). This relatively simple empirical criterion has its origins in Laplace's law for cylindrical tubes, which relates the vessel wall stress linearly to vessel diameter, predicting a linear increase in wall stress with increasing vessel (or aneurysm) diameter (Raghavan and Vorp 2000; Reeps et al. 2013; Vu et al. 2014; Polzer and Gasser 2015; Parikh et al. 2018).

Laplace's prediction is valid for uniform spherical or cylindrical shapes featuring a thin wall; however, AAAs present more complex curvature-based shapes with variable diameters and thicknesses throughout their geometry, hence rendering Laplace's law impractical and too simple for studying the mechanics of AAAs (Vu et al. 2014; Gharahi et al. 2015; Parikh et al. 2018). Additionally, recent studies have identified patients featuring maximal aneurysm diameters smaller than 5.5 cm, who nevertheless experienced rupture, and, conversely, patients featuring a $\boldsymbol{D_{max}}$ of 5.5 cm or larger, who have remained stable throughout their life (Tang et al. 2014; Gharahi et al. 2015; Shang, Nathan, and Woo 2015; Schmitz-Rixen, Keese, and Hakimi 2016; Parikh et al. 2018).

From a biomechanical point of view, rupture is the result of the mechanical failure of the aortic wall tissue (Stevens et al. 2017; Wittek et al. 2018). In a healthy aorta, the elastin and collagen network is linked with smooth muscle cells (SMC) allowing uniform mechanical properties throughout the entire length of the aorta. In aneurysmal tissue, the degradation of elastin and collagen fibers changes the stiffness and compliance of the tissue, causing localized heterogeneities in the mechanical properties, which further lead to non-uniform load bearing capacity throughout the AAA length (Wilson et al. 2003; Tierney, Callanan, and McGloughlin 2012; Wittek et al. 2018). Rupture happens when the overall effective stress experienced by the aneurysm wall exceeds the mechanical strength of the vessel tissue, now altered by the remodeling induced by disease (Fillinger et al. 2003; Wilson et al. 2003; Doyle et al. 2009; Wilson et al. 2017). As such, regions featuring compromised mechanical strength are therefore more susceptible to aneurysm formation and consequent rupture. Nevertheless, although the mechanical strength of the vessel wall cannot be non-invasively measured or quantified, regions experiencing higher stress than others are more likely to experience rupture. This theory has been foundational for the work by Fillinger et al., who revealed that peak wall stress (PWS) may serve as a more accurate biomechanical indicator of potential rupture (Fillinger et al. 2002).

While studies have shown that PWS has a significant correlation with D_{max}, it has also been proved that PWS correlates strongly with other parameters, such as geometrical (asymmetry, tortuosity, volume) (Martufi et al. 2009; Georgakarakos et al. 2010; Shum et al. 2011; Raut et al. 2013; Vu et al. 2014; Jalalahmadi, Linte, and Helguera 2017; Parikh et al. 2018; Urrutia et al. 2018; Wu et al. 2019), biomechanical (blood pressure, intraluminal thrombus, wall thickness) (Raghavan et al. 2006; Tierney, Callanan, and McGloughlin 2012; Reeps et al. 2013; Polzer and Gasser 2015; Raut, Liua, and Finol 2015 Mix et al. 2017; Farotto et al. 2018; Jalalahmadi-b et al. 2018; Tang et al. 2019; Wu et al. 2019;), and morphological parameters, which are related to the patient's life-style and health history (age, gender, health record, smoking status) (Chaikof et al. 2009; Raut et al. 2013; Karthikesalingam et al. 2014; Schmitz-Rixen, Keese, and Hakimi 2016; Villard and Hultgren 2018). Since PWS incorporates a much wider range of parameters affecting the AAA behavior besides D_{max}, it has been proposed as a more comprehensive and potentially more effective AAA rupture criterion than D_{max} alone, especially for aneurysms featuring a D_{max} smaller than 5.5 cm that are not deemed at risk according to the traditional clinical D_{max} criterion. However, AAAs are mostly asymptomatic, which means they might rupture at any time (Reeps et al. 2013). Notwithstanding all the studies and efforts to predict and prevent rupture, AAA remains the 12th leading cause of death in the United State (Polzer and Gasser 2015; Ramadan, Al-Omran, and Verma 2017). Accordingly, the estimation of rupture risk in a patient specific basis is the most problematic issue in clinical management (Martufi et al. 2009; Reeps et al. 2013).

MORPHOLOGY OF AAA

Main risk factors affecting this degenerative disease have been categorized in the following principal groups (Schmitz-Rixen, Keese, and Hakimi 2016; Vu et al. 2014):

1. *Geometrical parameters* summarize the overall geometry and shape of any individual AAA: 1D size parameters such as maximum transverse diameter (D_{max}), 2D shape parameters like asymmetry and tortuosity, 3D size parameters such as volume, and 3D shape parameters like 3D isoperimetric ratio and second-order curvature-based indices.
2. *Biomechanical parameters* study the effects of the biological factors on AAA: wall stress, intraluminal thrombus, and wall thickness.
3. *Demographical parameters* are related to lifestyle, habits and health history of each individual patient, such as age, gender, health record, and smoking etc.

It has been shown that each of these categories may increase the risk of AAA rupture at the end of its growth due to gradual wall weakening (Vu et al. 2014; Schmitz-Rixen, Keese, and Hakimi 2016; Wittek et al. 2018). As such, before we investigate influence of each of these parameter categories on AAA rupture risk and its behavior in more detail, a review of morphology of AAA will be presented.

As mentioned earlier, it was hypothesized that the main reason for the development of AAA is the increased weakening of the aortic wall due to the metabolic activity of the metalloproteinase matrix at the aneurysm site (Fillinger et al. 2003; Tang et al. 2014; Galarreta et al. 2017; Farotto et al. 2018). To this extent, this section serves as an overview of the main biological metabolic activities including inflammatory and degradation, transforming growth factor beta (TGF-β), presence of intraluminal thrombus, draped aorta and calcification occurring in the AAA site and affecting its growth and rupture (Vu et al. 2014; Wittek et al. 2018).

All aneurysms suffer from different degrees of inflammation and the degeneration of the connective tissue that makes up the aortic wall (elastin and collagen network), which, in turn, will alter the stiffness of the AAA wall. The different degree of inflammation can happen due to the presence of macrophages, lymphocytes and dendritic cells. These different types of white blood cells are responsible for the immune system of the arteries wall within the human body. Macrophage penetration increases harmful angiogenesis and lymph-angiogenesis within the vessel wall (Sano et al. 2014; Schmitz-Rixen, Keese, and Hakimi 2016). Meanwhile, growth of intravascular lymphatic vessels intensifies the secretion of pro-inflammatory cytokines from lymphocytes and monocytes (Zhou et al. 2011; Sano et al. 2014; Jalalzadeh, Indrakusuma, and Planken 2016; Schmitz-Rixen, Keese, and Hakimi 2016). It has been shown that the smooth muscle cells (SMC) in the AAA wall express a process of splitting elastin and other components of the extracellular matrix (ECM), inducing further ECM degradation and eventually vessel dilation and rupture (Egido 2011; Airhart et al. 2014; Michel, Martin-Ventura, and Niestrawska et al. 2016; Schmitz-Rixen, Keese, and Hakimi 2016; Stevens et al. 2017). Additionally, elastin and collagen degradation in the tunica media results in a remarkable structural deformation of the aortic wall, influencing the imbalance of the cellular and extracellular matrix homeostasis, causing the thinning and weakening of the aortic wall (Martufi et al. 2009). Matrix-Metallo-Proteinases (MMPs) are zinc- and calcium- based proteins that are responsible for the elastin and collagen degradation (Wang et al. 2013). While there is a minimum concentration of MMPs in a the normal aorta, it has been shown that impulsive blood clotting during the formation of intraluminal thrombus (ILT) is responsible for the activation of more MMPs at the AAA sac location (Raut et al. 2013).

Another biological factor affecting AAA formation and progression is the transforming growth factor beta (TGF-β), which is responsible for the regulation of fibroblast differentiation and induction of ECM deposition. It has been shown that TGF-β has a different impact on different embryonic origins of vascular smooth muscle cells (VSMC) (depending on their location throughout the aorta). TGF-β elevates VSMC growth in cells toward the thoracic aorta, and simultaneously prohibits VSMC growth in the abdominal aorta. Therefore, different embryonic origins result diametrically unsimilar roles of VSMCs in thoracic and abdominal aneurysms. Hence, it has been hypothesized that intensifying TGF-β signals could be used as a prevention or treatment approach for human AAAs (Wang et al. 2013; Schmitz-Rixen, Keese, and Hakimi 2016).

Intraluminal thrombus, which will be revisited in greater in detail in the Biomechanical Properties section, can also be considered as a preventing biological factor against rupture, since it increases the thickness of AAA, which, in turn, is inversely proportional to the wall stress distribution, and, consequently to its rupture, due to the role of the hoop stress. In reality, inherent metabolic activity within the thrombus reduces the aortic wall thickness, which increases the risk of rupture by producing an attenuation in intraluminal blood flow; this effect is referred to as hyper attenuation (Vu et al. 2014).

The loss of normal aorta wall convexity, called draped aorta, is another biological reason for AAA growth. This occurs when the normal fat layers between aneurysm and vertebra vanish. Therefore, the posterior wall of AAA will shape as the anterior surface of the vertebra, increasing the pressure, as well as the risk of rupture (Vu et al. 2014). Figure 2 shows an example of a patient-specific abdominal image featuring both ILT and a draped aorta.

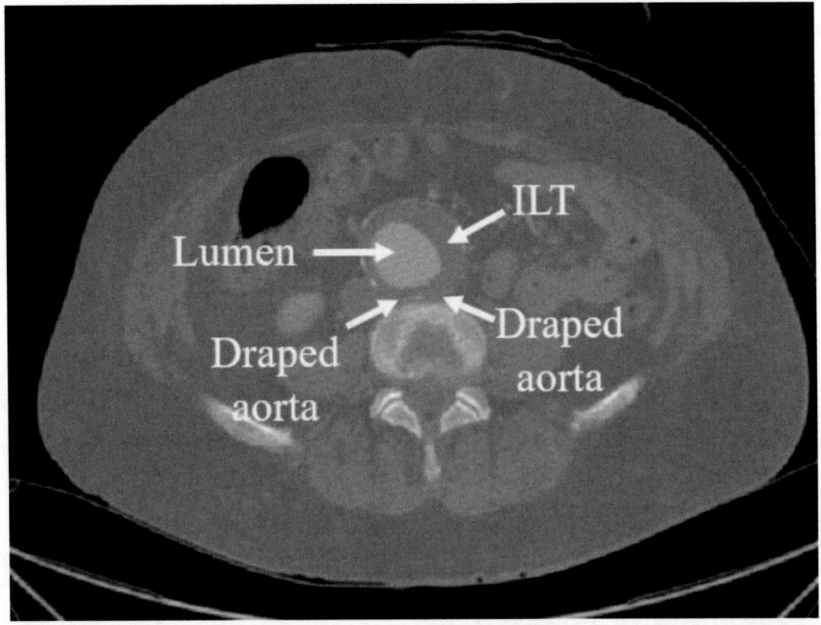

Figure 2. Axial enhanced CT image of AAA illustrating: ILT, the lumen of aorta, and the effect of draped aorta, where the posterior wall of aorta is being pushed against the anterior surface of the vertebral column

Calcification has been introduced as a sign of degenerative provocative process in the arterial wall (Bihari et al. 2013; Barretta et al. 2017). Using a mechanical tensile failure test, it was shown that calcified tissue showed a significantly higher failure probability than fibrous tissue, implying that calcification has an important impact on AAA rupture risk (Korte et al. 1997; Schmitz-Rixen, Keese, and Hakimi 2016), although there is no significant relation between the amount of calcification and the stress in AAA. However, calcification reduces the biomechanical stability of AAA by inducing a more mechanically more rigid structure, which makes it less resistant against the biomechanical stress caused by increasing blood pressure in the vessel (Korte et al. 1997; Barretta et al. 2017). This, in turn, increases the AAA rupture risk, which implies that the location of calcification in the AAA might have a greater effect on PWS than the amount of calcification (Bihari et al. 2013; Schmitz-Rixen, Keese, and Hakimi 2016).

PARAMETERS AFFECTING AAA: GEOMETRICAL INDICES

When monitoring patients with AAA overtime, it is necessary to prove that surgery and all related expenses compensate the mortality probability and prevent the risk of rupture. Today, the clinical criteria for elective repair of AAA are usually based on the maximum transverse diameter of AAA (with a critical value of $D_{max} > 5.5$ cm for men and $D_{max} > 5$ cm for women) and the growth rate of 1 cm per year (Vorp, Raghavan, and Webster 1998; Vu et al. 2014; Wanhainen, Mani, and Golledge 2016). These criteria follow Laplace's law, which implies a linear relation between diameter and wall tension in cylindrical tubes, meaning wall stress increases with an increase in the diameter of vessel (Raghavan and Vorp 2000; Reeps et al. 2013; Vu et al. 2014; Polzer and Gasser 2015).

However, it was indicated that relying only on D_{max} and rate of growth for clinical decision making is not sufficient, as in some cases, aneurysms with larger D_{max} do not rupture, while some smaller ones do. Moreover, Laplace's law fails due to the fact that AAAs have more complex shapes than simple cylinders (Raghavan and Vorp 2000; Reeps et al. 2013; Vu et al. 2014; Polzer and Gasser 2015). Also, solely considering D_{max} ignores other characteristics of each individual AAA, which are highly variable and may significantly affect AAA severity and rupture risk (Vorp, Raghavan, and Webster 1998). Meanwhile, it has been shown that a positive correlation among a set of geometrical indices representative of the overall AAA geometry can be considered as a more viable factor to predict AAA rupture (Martufi et al. 2009; Tang et al. 2014; Schmitz-Rixen, Keese, and Hakimi 2016; Jalalahmadi, Helguera, and Linte 2017; Urrutia et al. 2018).

Therefore, to study AAA more accurately, an overall geometry assessment of an AAA, which considers its entire shape and size, is necessary. Research has been conducted utilizing different clinical quality imaging data to reconstruct 2D and 3D models of AAA, estimate geometrical indices and their roles as indicators for the rupture (Fillinger et al. 2003;Martufi et al. 2009; Georgakarakos et al. 2010; Shum et al. 2011; Lee et al. 2013; Tang et al. 2014).

Fillinger et al. (Fillinger et al. 2003) statistically studied 2D computed tomography (CT) scans of AAA of multiple patients and investigated 40 different geometrical and demographical variables that were associated with AAA rupture. The studies concluded that both aneurysm diameter and tortuosity affect AAA rupture. Their study used manually segmented AAA geometries from 2D CT data, mainly because 3D CT data were not consistently available for all patients, as well as the low quality of some existing 3D CT images (Fillinger et al. 2003). In addition, Martufi et al. (Martufi et al. 2009) evaluated 25 geometrical parameters related to the shape and size of AAAs in a non-clinical case with the goal of estimating the overall geometry and fusiform degree of AAA. The authors developed a custom algorithm implemented in MATLAB that used CT data of nine un-ruptured AAAs to reconstruct their model. Their results illustrated that the patients with high risk of rupture were associated with a positive correlation between geometrical indices and wall thickness. Therefore, they concluded that a positive correlation between all geometrical indices and wall thickness should be considered as a more precise rupture risk indicator (Martufi et al. 2009).

In 2013 Tang et al. (Tang et al. 2014) conducted an additional study in which they evaluated 27 geometrical indices that may affect AAA rupture risk. In their work, CT scans from both symptomatic (symptomatic here refers to those patients who have been admitted to the hospital because they had pain and were ready for surgery) and asymptomatic AAA patients were used to reconstruct a 3D aneurysm model using MATLAB. The study claimed that gender, maximal diameter, and 14 other geometrical indices had a higher influence on the rupture risk (Tang et al. 2014) than D_{max} alone, as previously postulated. These geometrical indices, which were introduced by Fillinger et al. (Fillinger et al. 2003), Martufi et al. (Martufi et al. 2009) and Tang et al. (Tang et al. 2014), have been utilized by many other researchers to better understand the behavior of AAA and investigate more accurate methods for assessing AAA severity and probability of rupture (Georgakarakos et al. 2010; Shum et al. 2011; Zeinali-Davarani, Raguin, and Vorp 2011; Lee et al. 2013). The definitions of some of these indices are illustrated in Figure 3.

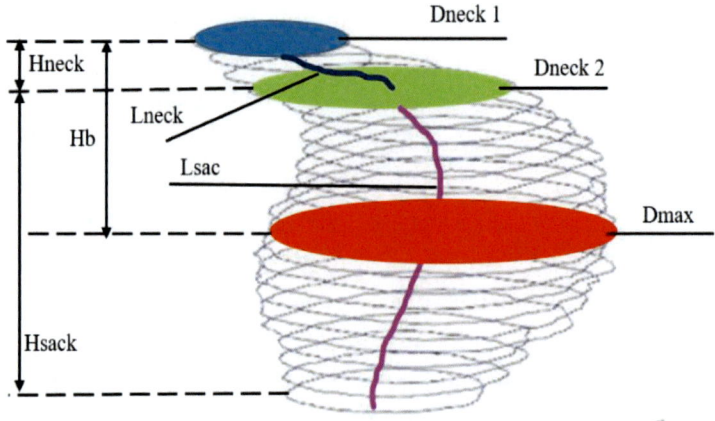

Figure 3. Schematic of sample AAA showing 1-dimensional geometrical indices introduced by Fillinger et al. 2003, Martufi et al. 2009, Tang et al. 2014 to study the AAA behavior.

Nevertheless, despite many investigations performed on geometrical indices and their effects on AAA's risk of rupture, there is still more to know about AAA and other potential parameters which might affect their behavior and rupture risk, especially for the case of ruptured AAAs that feature a D_{max} smaller than the critical D_{max}. As mentioned earlier, the growth of AAA happens when metabolic activities result in elastin and collagen fragmentation and degradation, which change the stiffness and consequently stress- and strain-bearing capacity of the AAA wall (Raghavan and Vorp 2000; Heng et al. 2008; Wilson, Baek, and Humphrey 2012). Moreover, most AAAs have different degrees of intraluminal thrombus (ILT) and localized calcification, both of which result in variable wall thickness along the length of AAA. These conditions contribute to the localized mechanical material properties in different regions of AAA leading to an uneven wall stress and strength distribution, reducing tolerance to high blood pressure levels that make the aneurysm more prone to rupture, leading to the death of patients (Raghavan and Vorp 2000; Speelman et al. 2007; Wilson, Baek, and Humphrey 2012; Powell 2014). Therefore, it is essential to consider the changes in biomechanical characteristics of the AAA wall tissue to generate comprehensive models that may predict rupture. In the next section we will discuss these concepts in more details.

PARAMETERS AFFECTING AAA: BIOMECHANICAL PARAMETERS

From a biomechanical point of view, the ultimate cause of AAA rupture is the exceedingly high aortic wall stress at the AAA site, higher than the vessel wall strength (Doyle et al. 2009; Leemans et al. 2017; Stevens et al. 2017; Wittek et al. 2018; Farotto et al. 2018). In Section 1.2, the biological phenomena which alter the normal aortic tissue were discussed. In this section, the major biomechanical parameters that have the potential to affect the AAA behavior and its rupture will be reviewed. These parameters include: material properties of aortic wall at the AAA bulge, wall thickness, intraluminal thrombus, and loading conditions. Investigating the AAA behavior and accurately assessing its risk of rupture entail the reconstruction of a 3D AAA model and the estimation of the developed peak wall stress in response to the loading conditions (i.e., internal blood pressure within the AAA), geometrical and biomechanical parameters.

Until recently, most AAA studies have been conducted under the assumption that modeling the aortic wall as a homogeneous material featuring linear elastic behavior may be sufficient (Vorp, Raghavan, and Muluk 1996; Elger et al. 1996; Vorp, Raghavan, and Webster 1998; Martino, Guadagni, and Fumero 2001; Georgakarakos et al. 2010). However, it has been acknowledged that the wall of the aorta has nonlinear elastic behavior, as many other soft biological tissues do (Patel et al. 1995; Fillinger et al. 2004; Georgakarakos et al. 2010; Shum et al. 2011). The collagen fibers that make up the different layers in the aortic wall are responsible for this non-linearity (Patel et al. 1995; Borghi et al. 2006; Shum et al. 2011; Wittek et al. 2018). Therefore, biomechanical models that do not consider the nonlinear elastic tissue properties may not be sufficiently accurate to mimic the actual stress–strain behavior of the aorta. Raghavan and Vorp (Raghavan and Vorp 2000) conducted a study in which 69 wall specimens of AAA patients were used to estimate the nonlinear elastic material properties of AAA wall. They proposed a two-parameter hyper-elastic, isotropic, incompressible material model (i.e., a special case of the generalized power law neo-Hookean model) to portray the mechanical behavior of the AAA wall. This model is described by two hyper-elastic material parameters with the mean values of $\alpha = 17.4 \pm 1.5$ N/cm^2 and $\mu = 188.1 \pm 37.2$ N/cm^2, where α represents bulk modulus, which is a measurement for deformation, and μ is a representative of shear modulus. Moreover, they reported less than 4% variation in wall stress in response to wall tissue parameter changes within the 95% confidence intervals. As such, if the actual patient-specific material properties are not available, their mean values may be used as the sufficiently reliable and viable parameters with 95% confidence (Raghavan and Vorp 2000).

Figure 4 illustrates one sample of the wall stress distribution with identification of PWS location. This distribution is generated using the authors' AAA computational model (Jalalahmadi, Helguera, and Linte 2017; Jalalahmadi-b et al. 2018).

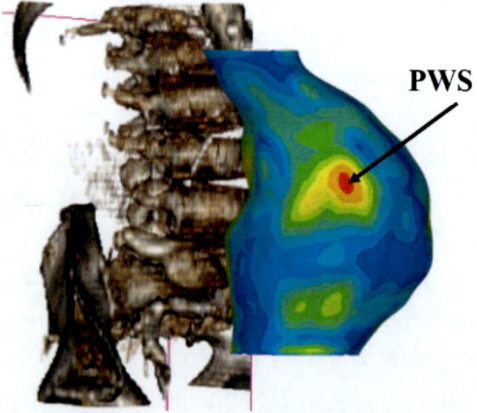

Figure 4. Distribution of the wall stress on the right posterior wall of a sample AAA. Black arrow shows the location of peak wall stress (PWS) at the inflection point.

In light of the different biological phenomena that contribute to the remodeling of the aortic wall that lead to the formation of AAAs (Section 1.2), it has become evident that the AAA wall tissue is better described by a heterogeneous model. Therefore, it was recently suggested that regional material properties may be more effective to describe AAA behavior rather than just assuming a uniform homogenous material property (either linear or hyper-elastic) for the whole AAA (Tierney, Callanan, and McGloughlin 2012; Wilson, Baek, and Humphrey 2012; Reeps et al. 2013; Mix et al. 2017). Wilson et al. (Wilson, Baek, and Humphrey 2012) studied the mechano-biological effects of ILT and regional damage in the extracellular matrix due to degradation that results in a regional anisotropic material stiffness and regional wall thickness, which need to be taken into account when studying AAA behavior and rupture risk. Their study showed that the stiffest aortic material tends to have a slower growth rate and lowest stretch in collagen fibers, while the least stiff aortas experienced the higher stress and higher expansion rates (Wilson, Baek, and Humphrey 2012).

Tierney et al. (Tierney, Callanan, and McGloughlin 2012) used CT images acquired at peak systole and end diastole, when the blood pressure is highest and lowest, respectively, depicting the AAA neck and D_{max} location to calculate the strain developed in the wall tissue, as well as, the elastic properties at the location of the neck and D_{max}. They showed that the location of PWS was similar for a homogenous AAA model and an AAA model featuring regional material properties. However, they concluded the strains predicted by the two models were different in magnitude by approximately 5%, which also resulted in different PWS values (Tierney, Callanan, and McGloughlin 2012). Similarly, Reeps et al. (Reeps et al. 2013) used AAA wall samples from 50 patients who underwent open surgery to measure several mechanical wall properties, including wall thickness, stiffness, wall strength, and failure tension. They showed that wall thickness is related to metabolic activity of the wall and also to the ILT. While failure tension showed a positive correlation with ILT, AAA volume, and wall thickness, wall strength has a strong inverse correlation with wall thickness. They concluded that to more accurately predict the rupture risk of AAA, all of these parameters have to be considered in the modeling procedure (Reeps et al. 2013). Limitations associated with these studies include: small sample size, use of idealized AAA geometries for simplicity, omission of the ILT effects, use of only partial CT images of AAA, consideration of only a limited number (four) of material regions for the entire AAA, collection of samples from patients who had undergone open surgery or repair (hence a small sample size), and use of PET/CT imaging for more accurate wall thickness prediction along with the metabolic activity at the site, even though this imaging method is not a standard clinical method for AAA and cannot be provided for a large sample size of patients (Tierney, Callanan, and McGloughlin 2012; Wilson, Baek, and Humphrey 2012; Reeps et al. 2013).

Meanwhile, it has been shown that the presence of intraluminal thrombus (ILT) impacts both aortic wall degeneration and PWS in the AAA (Stevens et al. 2017; Wittek et al. 2018). Figure 5 illustrates the ILT and the wall stress distribution for an AAA sample (Jalalahmadi-a et al. 2018; Jalalahmadi-b et al. 2018). ILT is a result of disturbed blood flow and blood stagnation in the AAA sac that could reach a thickness of 3 cm and more (Martufi et al. 2009; Achille, G. Tellides, and Humphrey 2016; Stevens et al. 2017). Previous studies illustrated that a larger D_{max} and thicker ILT were observed in ruptured AAAs in comparison to unruptured aneurysms, indicating a positive correlation between ILT and rupture risk (Martufi et al. 2009; Georgakarakos et al. 2010; Stevens et al. 2017). It has been pointed out that ILT makes a barrier for oxygen transfer and recreates a hypoxia environment between thrombus and AAA wall, especially at the site of thicker ILT, which increases inflammation of the wall and wall weakening by diminishing smooth muscle cells (SMCs) and extracellular matrix via proteolytic degradation of elastin and collagen (Michel, Martin-Ventura, and Egido 2011; Schmitz-Rixen, Keese, and Hakimi 2016; Stevens et al. 2017). This causes AAA wall thinning and consequently increases the risk of rupture (Schmitz-Rixen, Keese, and Hakimi 2016). However, the effect of ILT on PWS remains controversial and it has been recognized that a larger ILT is associated with higher AAA growth rate, while a lower wall stress is presented in the thicker parts of the wall against a higher wall stress in the thinner locations of the AAA wall (Speelman et al. 2007; Achille, G.

Tellides, and Humphrey 2016; Schmitz-Rixen, Keese, and Hakimi 2016; Stevens et al. 2017). The degeneration that occurs in the wall structure in the presence of AAA affects the mechanical characteristics; additionally, ILT has a softer tissue in comparison to AAA wall. This results in a more linear stress-strain relation for ILT compared to nonlinear stress-strain response for AAA wall, increasing the heterogeneous structure of AAA wall (Stevens et al. 2017; Wittek et al. 2018).

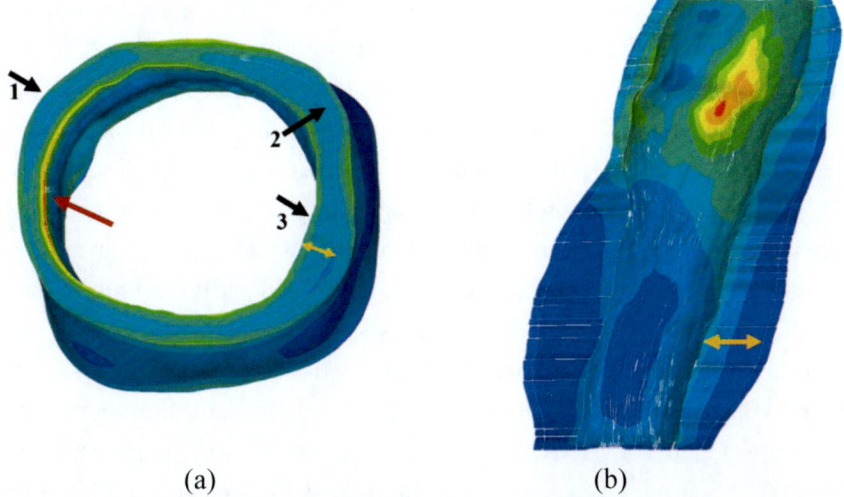

Figure 5. (a) An axial view of AAA with black arrow 1 showing outer wall, black arrow 2 showing inner wall, black arrow 3 showing the lumen wall (ILT lies between the inner wall and the lumen wall: yellow double-arrow), and red arrow indicating the location of PWS; (b) Coronal plane view of the wall stress distribution on the posterior wall of the AAA (yellow double-arrow indicating the ILT).

Furthermore, the response of the vessel wall to different loading conditions – typically internal pressure exerted by the blood flow inside the aneurysm – is in the form of internal stress and inherent deformation (or strain) (Raghavan and Vorp 2000; Wilson et al. 2003; Wanhainen, Mani, and Golledge 2016; Mix et al. 2017;). While the stress distribution developed within simple geometries may be estimated using analytical solutions, complex geometries, on the other hand, require numerical solutions, typically obtained using finite element analysis (FEA). The finite element method divides a complex geometry into a finite number of small elements, where a higher number of elements with smaller size for each individual element give a more accurate solution. FEA can be used to generate a stress contour for each individual AAA and provides a reliable and noninvasive clinical way to monitor influence of different parameters on the stress distribution of a single AAA (Raghavan and Vorp 2000; Doyle et al. 2009; Polzer and Gasser 2015; Wanhainen, Mani, and Golledge 2016; Leemans et al. 2017; Biehler and Wall 2018).

Vorp et al. (Vorp, Raghavan, and Webster 1998) used Pro-Engineer V16.0™ to model the virtual AAAs for their study and conducted a FEA using ANSYS™ for the first time in AAA studies, to determine the effects of maximal diameter D_{max} and AAA asymmetry on the overall effective wall stress. Their numerical study assumed homogeneous and linear elastic vessel wall properties and concluded that the peak wall stress increased with increasing maximal diameter and AAA asymmetry (Vorp, Raghavan, and Webster 1998). Even though their study had a handful of limitations, including the assumption of homogeneous and linear elastic vessel wall properties, use of 3D synthetic models constructed with an in-house MATLAB algorithm, uniform wall thickness and mechanical properties for the entire length of AAA, it was a start for a more comprehensive characterization of AAA. Since then, the use of FEA made it possible for researchers to incorporate the effects of biomechanical and biological phenomena in order to more accurately investigate AAA behavior, rupture and possible dogmatic and treatment methods in a patient specific way (Heng et al. 2008; Doyle et al. 2009; Joldes et al. 2016; Leemans et al. 2017; Biehler and Wall 2018; Wittek et al. 2018).

So far, we have learned that biomechanical factors affect the AAA formation and its rupture through changes in the biological characteristics of the vessel wall. These factors, along with associated geometrical parameters, have been the main focus when studying numerical approaches to assess AAA severity and predict AAA rupture more precisely. However, it has been shown that personal health conditions, family history, and life-style patterns might be related to the origin of the evolving biological phenomena that contribute to the formation and growth of AAAs. Hence, in the following section, we will briefly review these aspects.

PARAMETERS AFFECTING AAA: DEMOGRAPHICAL PARAMETERS

It has been shown that family history, health record, and other demographical parameters (age and gender) influence AAA and its behavior (Fillinger et al. 2003; Björck and Wanhainen 2013; Rudarakanchana and Powell 2013; Villard and Hultgren 2018). Family history is one of the genetic parameters, which can affect the chance of getting AAA. It was shown that a first generation relative of patients who have had AAA are at an increased risk of developing an AAA; however, this chance can differ from 1% to 30% (Björck and Wanhainen 2013). On the other hand, since there is no uniform method to investigate family history, and most studies have only been based on questionnaires, the effect of family history on AAA remains controversial (Björck and Wanhainen 2013).

Smoking can be assumed as the main environmental risk factor for AAA as a degenerative disorder (Björck and Wanhainen 2013; Robert, Juillière, and Gabet 2017). In a study that, accounted for all other risk factors, it was shown that 71% of AAA patients were smokers. However, due to the fact that there are fewer people that smoke and better cardiovascular care, especially in developed countries, the mortality rate is decreasing (Chaikof et al. 2009; Björck and Wanhainen 2013; Rudarakanchana and Powell 2013). This also affects the age when the repair is performed for patients with AAA. Due to fewer people smoking, the age at the time of repair has increased from 65, when men start being screened for AAA, to 74 in different countries (Rudarakanchana and Powell 2013; Takagi, Ando, and Umemoto 2017).

Women consistently display lower presence of AAA than men in the same age range. However, the rate of the rupture and consequently the rate of mortality in women is higher than in men (Björck and Wanhainen 2013; Engelberger et al. 2017; Robert, Juillière, and Gabet 2017; Takagi, Ando, and Umemoto 2017; Villard and Hultgren 2018). Therefore, The Society for Vascular Surgery (SVS) in USA suggested that women 65 years of age or older, who have smoked at any time in their life or have a family history of AAA, are recommended for ultrasound imaging screening (Reeps et al. 2013; Vu et al. 2014).

Diet and obesity have been identified as other demographical parameters that can affect AAA (Björck and Wanhainen 2013). Two of the most significant parameters related to them are diabetes and chronic kidney disease (CKD) (Björck and Wanhainen 2013; Reeps et al. 2013). It has been demonstrated that diabetes shows a positive correlation with wall thickness, while a negative correlation between wall thickness and patients who suffer from the chronic kidney disease (CKD) was observed (Reeps et al. 2013).

Therefore, to have a comprehensive understanding about AAA and potential monitoring and treatment methods, incorporation of all three main categories of parameters, namely, geometrical, biomechanical, and morphological parameters in a predictive model is essential (Martufi et al. 2009; Speelman et al. 2010; Rudarakanchana and Powell 2013; Karthikesalingam et al. 2014; Schmitz-Rixen, Keese, and Hakimi 2016). To do so, imaging of AAA patients has become increasingly useful, in the effort to better understand patient specific anatomy, as well as potentially reduce the rate of mortality by better planning the interventional procedure for those in need of surgical repair (Patel et al. 1995; Galarreta et al. 2017). In the next section we will discuss different imaging modalities for AAA imagery.

IMAGING METHODS

Due to reduced smoking and better health care, the age at the time of repair for patients with AAA is increasing worldwide (Rudarakanchana and Powell 2013; Takagi, Ando, and Umemoto 2017). It has been suggested to start monitoring cardiovascular diseases including AAA (Rudarakanchana and Powell 2013; Sprynger et al. 2019) for patients 65 years or older. Using ultrasonography, a maximal transverse diameter greater or equal to 3.00 cm has been used as the criterion to justify a follow-up for patients

(Rudarakanchana and Powell 2013; Engelberger et al. 2017; Iwakoshi, Hirai, and Kichikawa 2019). For a patient with an AAA diameter up to 4.5 cm, 3-year follow-up intervals are recommended and once the D_{max} reaches 5.0 cm, annual follow-ups are recommended; moreover, in the event of further increase in D_{max}, a 6-month follow-up frequency has been suggested (Rudarakanchana and Powell 2013; Engelberger et al. 2017; Sprynger et al. 2019).

Comparatively low cost (relative to Computed Tomography Angiography (CTA) and Magnetic Resonance Imaging (MRI)), easy accessibility, and no ionizing radiation exposure have contributed to Ultrasonography (US) becoming the common screening method for AAA (Wanhainen, Mani, and Golledge 2016; Liisberg, Diederichsen, and Lindholt 2017; Iwakoshi, Hirai, and Kichikawa 2019; Sprynger et al. 2019). Two-dimensional (2D) US can be used to perform a simple diameter measurement and assessment of wall motion, while three-dimensional (3D) US may supply additional information on AAA morphology or geometry (Rudarakanchana and Powell 2013; Sprynger et al. 2019). However, the clinically imposed limitation on intra-observer variability of 27 mm and inter-observer variability of 2-10 mm (intra-observer measurements for D_{max} show a variability of 27 mm between 4 different observers where the results showed a 27 mm variability between the min and max of those measurements), makes US a less accurate and viable method, especially in the case of a clinical decision-making process, while CT and MRI both show intra- and inter-observer variability of less than 2 mm (Rudarakanchana and Powell 2013; Wanhainen, Mani, and Golledge 2016).

On the other hand, computed tomography angiography (CTA) produces more detailed information on AAA geometry (length, volume and so on, rather than just D_{max}) and morphology (ILT presence) with advanced 3D image reconstruction and estimation of the entire vessel structure. These benefits over US imaging render Computed Tomography (CT) as the current standard pre-operative imaging method for AAA imaging. However, CT exposes patients to significant levels of radiation, which along with the risk of nephrogenic injuries constitute two of the down-sides of CTA

(Kauffmann et al. 2011; Rudarakanchana and Powell 2013; Liisberg, Diederichsen, and Lindholt 2017).

Magnetic Resonance Imaging (MRI) can be introduced as the best screening method for soft-tissue imaging with no radiation exposure and equally as good as CTA in providing details on AAA. MRI may provide information on morphological and mechanical aspects of AAA such as aortic wall decomposition and cellular activity (Jalalzadeh, Indrakusuma, and Planken 2016; Wanhainen, Mani, and Golledge 2016). However, it is expensive, and, therefore, not readily available for AAA screening in most medical centers (Rudarakanchana and Powell 2013; Wanhainen, Mani, and Golledge 2016).

Overall, ultrasonography imaging, thanks to its non-invasiveness, wide availability, and affordability remains the most popular imaging method of AAAs for diagnosis and follow-up (Rudarakanchana and Powell 2013; Wanhainen, Mani, and Golledge 2016; Liisberg, Diederichsen, and Lindholt 2017; Iwakoshi, Hirai, and Kichikawa 2019; Sprynger et al. 2019). Meanwhile, the use of CT imaging systems is growing as a more viable imaging modality for AAA, mainly due to their superior image quality and ability for 3D characterization and visualization, as well as their increased availability and affordability over the MRI systems (Liisberg, Diederichsen, and Lindholt 2017; Takagi, Ando, and Umemoto 2017).

TREATMENT METHODS

Currently, there is no pharmacological treatment to reduce growth or rupture risk of AAA (Wanhainen, Mani, and Golledge 2016; Locham et al. 2017). Standard treatments consist of either open or endovascular aneurysm surgical repair for patients with $D_{max} \geq 5.5$ cm (Wanhainen, Mani, and Golledge 2016; Locham et al. 2017; Nilsson, Hultgren, and Letterstål 2017; Holden 2018). For patients with symptomatic AAA, urgent treatment is required, which indicates appropriate pre-operative management and repair have to be done within 4 to 24 hours of admission. However, for a patient with an acute AAA, an immediate treatment is necessary (Vu et al. 2014;

Locham et al. 2017). If rupture happens, 50% of patients will die before arriving to the emergency room; moreover, there is up to 80% risk of mortality for patients undergoing AAA repair surgery 30 days post-procedure (Niestrawska et al. 2016; Barretta et al. 2017; Leemans et al. 2017; Wilson et al. 2017). In this section a brief explanation for each of treatment methods will be provided, along with their main characterizations.

Open Repair (OR)

The standard treatment for AAA is open abdominal surgery which demands a large-scale abdominal incision, clamping of the proximal abdominal aorta, and suturing of a graft that excludes the aneurysm (Vu et al. 2014; Locham et al. 2017). The most important advantage of open repair is rapid, secure, and effective control of proximal aorta and reduction of blood loss (Lee, Bae, and Chung 2015; Locham et al. 2017). Proximal control is performed by balloon occlusion which could be injected directly through the aorta or under fluoroscopic image guidance help through femoral or brachial artery (Lee, Bae, and Chung 2015; Locham et al. 2017).

Endovascular Aneurysm Repair (EVAR)

EVAR was first introduced in 1991 (Koncar et al. 2012; Williams and Brooke 2017). Using an endovascular technique, a covered stent-graft connects the proximal neck of the AAA to either one (mono-iliac stent graft) or both iliac arteries (bifurcated stent graft) to seclude the aortic wall from the normal arterial blood pressure (Vu et al. 2014; Piazza et al. 2017; Holden 2018). Figure 6 shows a schematic representation of EVAR. It was illustrated that EVAR could be useful in emergency situations, such as the repair of an acute AAA. It should be noted that not all patients are eligible for EVAR due to the fact that a stent-graft size and selection procedure are required to be adopted with patient anatomy. In some cases, this could lead to an expensive procedure, both logistically and financially. Pre-operative imaging of the AAA, as well as femoral and iliac artery anatomy, are needed in order to capture the suitable anatomical structure for EVAR procedure. Some challenging anatomical features include sufficient proximal neck length (more than 10-15 mm), normal proximal and distal neck diameters (less than 32 mm), limited neck angulation (between 60 to 90 degrees), a limited amount of mural thrombus and calcification (occupying less than 50% of the aortic circumference), sufficiently small iliac arteries (less than 5 mm diameter), or severe occlusive disease which might exclude the EVAR probability (Vu et al. 2014; Locham et al. 2017).

Additionally, EVAR is related to endoleaks, which are the main long-term uptakes of EVAR and might result in long-term AAA rupture (Vu et al. 2014; Kim et al. 2019; Orgera et al. 2019). To prevent endoleaks, CT imaging at 1 to 12 months after EVAR is suggested, followed by an annual monitoring program (Chaikof et al. 2009; Vu et al. 2014). In case of observing an endoleak in a follow-up screening, it is important to know its type, as each type requires a specific management strategy. In general, there are 4 categories of endoleaks:

1. Type I: Sealing zone endoleak
2. Type II: Retrograde flow from a covered aortic branch endoleak
3. Type III: Graft failure endoleak
4. Vendoleak or endotension; progression of the AAA diameter with no detectable endoleak on a dual phase.

Type I and III should be instantly addressed since they are considered equivalent to an untreated AAA (Vu et al. 2014; Orgera et al. 2019). Type II are more common and are not as life-threatening as the other 2 types. A 6-month follow-up is suggested for type II endoleaks, and, if any sign of aneurysm growth has been observed, an EVAR re-intervention is needed. In case of a Vendoleak, which occurs in up to 40% of patients who underwent EVAR (Vu et al. 2014; Williams and Brooke 2017; Kim et al. 2019), close imaging follow-up and open surgery constitute standard clinical management.

Another criterion to compare these two treatment methods – open repair vs. endovascular repair - is the average time of hospitalization, which amounts to 3 days on average for EVAR and 7 days for OR patients. However, patients who experienced EVAR are recommended to have a life-long follow-up due to higher risk of endoleaks than OR-treated patients (Piazza et al. 2017; Williams and Brooke 2017).

Unfortunately, because of the differences in interventional experience levels amongst physicians, anatomical inclusion criteria for EVAR still vary widely amongst medical centers, with eligibility rates ranging from 34 to 100% (Harkin et al. 2007; Vu et al. 2014). As a result, the selection of best treatment method remains widely dependent on the physician's decision and patient agreement (Harkin et al. 2007; Vu et al. 2014; Locham et al. 2017).

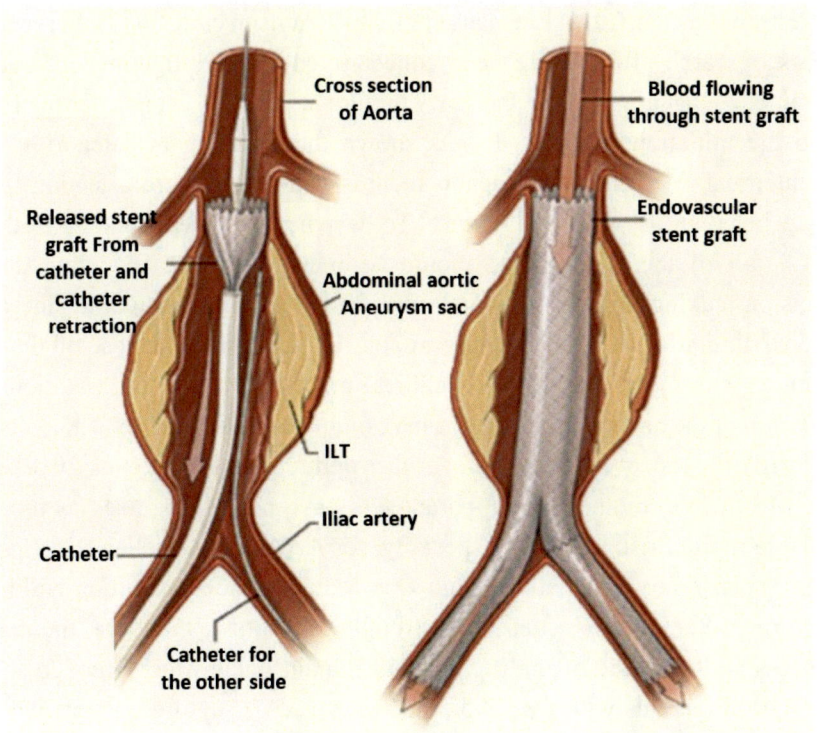

Figure 6. Schematic representation of endovascular aneurysm repair (EVAR) for abdominal aortic aneurysm (AAA) treatment.

CONCLUSION

In this chapter a comprehensive review of abdominal aortic aneurysm (AAA) physiology and behavior was presented. An overview of different geometrical, biomechanical and morphological parameters that affect AAA was provided. Also, various modeling techniques, imaging-based screening and follow-up methods, and different treatment strategies to investigate and deal with AAA were reviewed.

AAA is becoming one of the top tenth causes of death worldwide, with a mortality rate of 85-90% (Kazimierczak et al. 2019; Leach et al. 2019; Polzer et al. 2019). Moreover, while timely surgical repair is the preferred treatment approach, the risk of mortality for patients undergoing AAA repair surgery could be as high as 80% within 30 days of the procedure (Niestrawska et al. 2016; Leemans et al. 2017; Wilson et al. 2017). In recent years, research efforts have been concentrated on investigating different parameters that might affect the AAA rupture and help to get a better insight into the initiation of AAA. It was shown that three main categories of geometrical, biomechanical, health records and lifestyle are affecting the AAA behavior as well as its rupture. To have a better understanding of the AAA, all of these categories should be included in the modeling and decision-making process of course in different extends. However, due to ethical limitations as well as unavailable clinical trial on most of these features, currently, even the best clinical practices rely on the traditional criterion of the aneurysm transverse maximum diameter (i.e., D_{max} >5.5 cm) to justify the risk of intervention over the rupture risk (Polzer et al. 2019).

Meanwhile, biomechanical parameters have been recognized as more reliable rupture risk indicators, specially, for AAAs with smaller D_{max} (less than 5.5 cm). For most patients with D_{max} > 5.5 cm the intervention will be performed before they actually go through the rupture, therefore, the real process and outcome of the rupture will remain unknown. Moreover, the number of patients with D_{max} < 5.5 cm whose AAA ruptured, is relatively low, which makes it more challenging to study the effects of biomechanical parameters (Polzer et al. 2019). However, uncertainty about biomechanical factors arises from low availability of patient-specific material properties and wall strength of AAA wall tissue (Kazimierczak et al. 2019; Polzer et al. 2019). Most of the modeling research on AAA are image-based analysis which rely on computed tomography (CT) images. However, heterogeneity of the AAA wall and ILT are not traceable through CT; whilst MRI is able to resolve this issue, it is very costly and not affordable for many clinics (Leach et al. 2019). Therefore, despite increasing attention toward studying the regional material properties of the wall, the inclusion of material heterogeneity remains as a challenging limitation for most studies (Leach et al. 2019; Polzer et al. 2019).

Even though endovascular aneurysm repair (EVAR) is remarkably less invasive with a lower rate of mortality compared to open surgery, the need of a long-term imaging monitoring, to prevent post-operative complications, makes it more complicated (Kazimierczak et al. 2019; O'Donnell, Landon, and Schermerhorn 2019; Rouet et al. 2019; Orgera et al. 2019). Patient-specific stent grafts are coming more into attention to reduce the complexity of EVAR post-operative. Despite all the ongoing efforts in this area, incorporating of patient-specific ILT, overall geometry of AAA, chance of migration, infection, post-operative enlargement of stent graft, and most importantly endoleaks are some of the challenges to be resolved in the future (Kazimierczak et al. 2019; Kim et al. 2019; O'Donnell, Landon, and Schermerhorn 2019; Orgera et al. 2019).

As more patients are going through more frequent screening programs, more patients - who underwent EVAR repair - go more often for individually screening follow-ups, and due to reduction in smoking (Kazimierczak et al. 2019; O'Donnell, Landon, and Schermerhorn 2019; Rouet et al. 2019; Sprynger et al. 2019), mortality rate of AAA has been decreasing over the past decade. Nevertheless, there are still many people at risk of developing AAA and therefore, any research and development to prevent and repair AAA, mainly in a patient-specific manner, will not only save many lives, but also increase the patients' general health conditions and life expectancy. This could be achieved by increasing patient-specific investigations and clinical trial-based studies.

REFERENCES

Achille, P. D., Tellides, G. and Humphrey, J. D. (2016). Hemodynamics-driven deposition of intraluminal thrombus in abdominal aortic aneurysms. *International Journal for Numerical Methods in Biomedical Engineering*, *33*(5). doi: 10.1002/cnm.2828

Airhart, N. D., Brownstein, B., Schierding, W., Cobb, P., Arif, B., Ennis, T, Thompson R. W. Curci, J. A. (2013). Smooth Muscle Cells from Abdominal Aortic Aneurysms Are Unique and Can Independently and Synergistically Degrade Insoluble Elastin. *Journal of Vascular Surgery*, *57*(5). doi: 10.1016/j.jvs.2013.02.075

Barrett, H., Cunnane, E., Brien, J. O., Moloney, M., Kavanagh, E. and Walsh, M. (2017). On the effect of computed tomography resolution to distinguish between abdominal aortic aneurysm wall tissue and calcification: A proof of concept. *European Journal of Radiology*, *95*, 370–377. doi: 10.1016/j.ejrad.2017.08.023

Biehler, J. and Wall, W. A. (2017). The impact of personalized probabilistic wall thickness models on peak wall stress in abdominal aortic aneurysms. *International Journal for Numerical Methods in Biomedical Engineering*, *34*(2). doi: 10.1002/cnm.2922

Bihari, P., Shelke, A., Nwe, T., Mularczyk, M., Nelson, K., Schmandra, T., Knez P., Schmitz-Rixen, T. (2013). Strain Measurement of Abdominal Aortic Aneurysm with Real-time 3D Ultrasound Speckle Tracking. *European Journal of Vascular and Endovascular Surgery*, *45*(4), 315–323. doi: 10.1016/j.ejvs.2013.01.004

Björck, M. and Wanhainen, A. (2013). Pathophysiology of AAA: Heredity vs Environment. *Progress in Cardiovascular Diseases*, *56*(1), 2–6. doi: 10.1016/j.pcad.2013.05.003

Bogunovic, N., Meekel, J. P., Micha, D., Blankensteijn, J. D., Hordijk, P. L. and Yeung, K. K. (2019). Impaired smooth muscle cell contractility as a novel concept of abdominal aortic aneurysm pathophysiology. *Scientific Reports*, *9*(1). doi: 10.1038/s41598-019-43322-3

Borghi, A., Wood, N. B., Mohiaddin, R. H. and Xu, X. Y. (2006). 3D geometric reconstruction of thoracic aortic aneurysms. *Biomed Eng Online* 5:59. doi: 10.1186/1475-925X-5-59.

Chaikof, E. L., Brewster, D. C., Dalman, R. L., Makaroun, M. S., Illig, K. A., Sicard, G. A., Timaran C. H., Upchurch G. R., Veith, F. J. (2009). The care of patients with an abdominal aortic aneurysm: The Society for Vascular Surgery practice guidelines. *Journal of Vascular Surgery*, 50(4). doi: 10.1016/j.jvs.2009.07.002

Doyle, B. J., Callanan, A., Walsh, M. T., Grace, P. A. and Mcgloughlin, T. M. (2009). A Finite Element Analysis Rupture Index (FEARI) as an Additional Tool for Abdominal Aortic Aneurysm Rupture Prediction. *Vascular Disease Prevention*, 6(1), 114–121. doi: 10.2174/1567270000906010114

Figueiredo, G. N. D., Müller-Peltzer, K., Schwarze, V., Rübenthaler, J. and Clevert, D.-A. (2019). Ultrasound and contrast enhanced ultrasound imaging in the diagnosis of acute aortic pathologies. *Vasa*, 48(1), 17–22. doi: 10.1024/0301-1526/a000758

Elger, D. F., Blackketter, D. M., Budwig, R. S. and Johansen, K. H. (1996). The Influence of Shape on the Stresses in Model Abdominal Aortic Aneurysms. *Journal of Biomechanical Engineering*, 118(3), 326–332. doi: 10.1115/1.2796014

Engelberger S., Rossoa R., Sartib M., Del Grandec F., Canevascinia R., van den Berga J. C., Prousea G., and Giovannaccia L. (2017). Ultrasound screening for abdominal aortic aneurysms. (2017). *Swiss Medical Weekly*, 147(0910). doi: 10.4414/smw.2017.14412

Farotto, D., Segers, P., Meuris, B., Sloten, J. V. and Famaey, N. (2018). The role of biomechanics in aortic aneurysm management: requirements, open problems and future prospects. *Journal of the Mechanical Behavior of Biomedical Materials*, 77, 295–307. doi: 10.1016/j.jmbbm.2017.08.019

Fillinger, M. F., Raghavan, M., Marra, S. P., Cronenwett, J. L. and Kennedy, F. E. (2002). In vivo analysis of mechanical wall stress and abdominal aortic aneurysm rupture risk. *Journal of Vascular Surgery*, 36(3), 589–597. doi: 10.1067/mva.2002.125478.

Fillinger, M. F., Marra, S. P., Raghavan, M. and Kennedy, F. E. (2003). Prediction of rupture risk in abdominal aortic aneurysm during observation: Wall stress versus diameter. *Journal of Vascular Surgery*, *37*(4), 724–732. doi: 10.1067/mva.2003.213

Fillinger, M. F., Racusin, J., Baker, R. K., Cronenwett, J. L., Teutelink, A., Schermerhorn, M. L., Rzucidlo, E. M. (2004). Anatomic characteristics of ruptured abdominal aortic aneurysm on conventional CT scans: implications for rupture risk. *Journal of Vascular Surgery*, *39*(6), 1243–1252. doi: 10.1016/j.jvs.2004.02.025

Georgakarakos, E., Ioannou, C., Kamarianakis, Y., Papaharilaou, Y., Kostas, T., Manousaki, E. and Katsamouris, A. (2010). The Role of Geometric Parameters in the Prediction of Abdominal Aortic Aneurysm Wall Stress. *European Journal of Vascular and Endovascular Surgery*, *39*(1), 42–48. doi: 10.1016/j.ejvs.2009.09.026.

Gharahi, H., Zambrano, B., Lim, C., Choi, J., Lee, W. and Baek, S. (2015). On growth measurements of abdominal aortic aneurysms using maximally inscribed spheres. *Medical Engineering & Physics*, *37*(7), 683–691. doi: 10.1016/j.medengphy.2015.04.011.

Harkin, D., Dillon, M., Blair, P., Ellis, P. and Kee, F. (2007). Endovascular Ruptured Abdominal Aortic Aneurysm Repair (EVRAR): A Systematic Review. *Journal of Vascular Surgery*, *46*(6), 1309. doi: 10.1016/j.jvs.2007.09.054.

Heng, M. S., Fagan, M. J., Collier, J. W., Desai, G., Mccollum, P. T. and Chetter, I. C. (2008). Peak wall stress measurement in elective and acute abdominal aortic aneurysms. *Journal of Vascular Surgery*, *47*(1), 17–22. doi: 10.1016/j.jvs.2007.09.002

Holden, A. (2018). Aneurysm Repair with Endovascular Aneurysm Sealing Technique, Patient Selection, and Management of Complications. *Techniques in Vascular and Interventional Radiology*, *21*(3), 181–187. doi: 10.1053/j.tvir.2018.06.008.

Iwakoshi, S., Hirai, T. and Kichikawa, K. (2019). Updates on Ultrasonography Imaging in Abdominal Aortic Aneurysm. *Annals of Vascular Diseases*, *12*(3), 319–322. doi: 10.3400/avd.ra.19-00070

Jalalahmadi, G., Linte, C. and Helguera, M. (2017). A numerical framework for studying the biomechanical behavior of abdominal aortic aneurysm. *Medical Imaging 2017: Biomedical Applications in Molecular, Structural, and Functional Imaging.* doi: 10.1117/12.2254528.

Jalalahmadi-a, G., Helguera, M., Linte, C. A. and Mix, D. S. (2018). Toward modeling the effects of regional material properties on the wall stress distribution of abdominal aortic aneurysms. *Medical Imaging 2018: Biomedical Applications in Molecular, Structural, and Functional Imaging.* doi: 10.1117/12.2294558.

Jalalahmadi-b, G., Helguera, M., Mix, D. S., Hodis, S., Richards, M. S., Stoner, M. C. and Linte, C. A. (2018). (Peak) Wall Stress as An Indicator Of Abdominal Aortic Aneurysm Severity. *2018 IEEE Western New York Image and Signal Processing Workshop (WNYISPW).* doi: 10.1109/wnyipw.2018.8576453.

Jalalzadeh, H., Indrakusuma, R., Planken, R., Legemate, D., Koelemay, M. and Balm, R. (2016). Inflammation as a Predictor of Abdominal Aortic Aneurysm Growth and Rupture: A Systematic Review of Imaging Biomarkers. *European Journal of Vascular and Endovascular Surgery, 52*(3), 333–342. doi: 10.1016/j.ejvs.2016.05.002.

Joldes, G. R., Miller, K., Wittek, A. and Doyle, B. (2016). A simple, effective and clinically applicable method to compute abdominal aortic aneurysm wall stress. *Journal of the Mechanical Behavior of Biomedical Materials, 58,* 139–148. doi: 10.1016/j.jmbbm.2015.07.029.

Karthikesalingam, A., Holt, P. and Vidal-Diez, A. (2014). Mortality from Ruptured Abdominal Aortic Aneurysms: Clinical Lessons from a Comparison of Outcomes in England and the USA. *Journal of Vascular Surgery, 60*(1), 265–266. doi: 10.1016/j.jvs.2014.05.037

Kauffmann, C., Tang, A., Dugas, A., Therasse, É. Oliva, V. and Soulez, G. (2011). Clinical validation of a software for quantitative follow-up of abdominal aortic aneurysm maximal diameter and growth by CT angiography. *European Journal of Radiology, 77*(3), 502–508. doi: 10.1016/j.ejrad.2009.07.027

Kazimierczak, W., Serafin, Z., Kazimierczak, N., Ratajczak, P., Leszczyński, W., Bryl, Ł. and Lemanowicz, A. (2019). Contemporary imaging methods for the follow-up after endovascular abdominal aneurysm repair: a review. *Videosurgery and Other Miniinvasive Techniques*, *14*(1), 1–11. doi: 10.5114/wiitm.2018.78973

Kim H. O., Yim N. Y., Kim J. K., Kang Y. J., and Lee B. C. (2019). Endovascular Aneurysm Repair for Abdominal Aortic Aneurysm: A Comprehensive Review. *Korean J Radiol* 20 (8):1247-1265. doi: 10.3348/kjr.2018.0927.

Koncar I., Tolić M., Ilić N., Cvetković S., Dragas M., Cinara I., Kostić D., and Davidović L. (2012). Endovascular aortic repair: first twenty years. *Srp Arh Celok Lek* 140 (11-12):792-9.

Korte, C. L. D., Céspedes, E., Steen, A. F. V. D. and Lancée, C. T. (1997). Intravascular elasticity imaging using ultrasound: Feasibility studies in phantoms. *Ultrasound in Medicine & Biology*, *23*(5), 735–746. doi: 10.1016/s0301-5629(97)00004-5

Leach, J. R., Kao, E., Zhu, C., Saloner, D. and Hope, M. D. (2019). On the Relative Impact of Intraluminal Thrombus Heterogeneity on Abdominal Aortic Aneurysm Mechanics. *Journal of Biomechanical Engineering*, *141*(11). doi: 10.1115/1.4044143

Lee C. W., Bae M., and Chung W. S. (2015). General considerations of ruptured abdominal aortic aneurysm: ruptured abdominal aortic aneurysm. *Korean J Thorac Cardiovasc Surg* 48 (1):1-6. doi: 10.5090/kjtcs.2015.48.1.1.

Lee, K., Zhu, J., Shum, J., Zhang, Y., Muluk, S. C., Chandra, A. and Finol, E. A. (2012). Surface Curvature as a Classifier of Abdominal Aortic Aneurysms: A Comparative Analysis. *Annals of Biomedical Engineering*, *41*(3), 562–576. doi: 10.1007/s10439-012-0691-4

Leemans, E. L., Willems, T. P., Laan, M. J. V. D., Slump, C. H. and Zeebregts, C. J. (2016). Biomechanical Indices for Rupture Risk Estimation in Abdominal Aortic Aneurysms. *Journal of Endovascular Therapy*, *24*(2), 254–261. doi: 10.1177/1526602816680088

Liisberg, M., Diederichsen, A. C. and Lindholt, J. S. (2017). Abdominal ultrasound scanning versus non-contrast computed tomography as screening method for abdominal aortic aneurysm – a validation study from the randomized DANCAVAS study. *BMC Medical Imaging*, *17*(1). doi: 10.1186/s12880-017-0186-8

Locham, S., Lee, R., Nejim, B., Aridi, H. D. and Malas, M. (2017). Mortality after endovascular versus open repair of abdominal aortic aneurysm in the elderly. *Journal of Surgical Research*, *215*, 153–159. doi: 10.1016/j.jss.2017.03.061

Martino, E. D., Guadagni, G., Fumero, A., Ballerini, G., Spirito, R., Biglioli, P. and Redaelli, A. (2001). Fluid–structure interaction within realistic three-dimensional models of the aneurysmatic aorta as a guidance to assess the risk of rupture of the aneurysm. *Medical Engineering & Physics*, *23*(9), 647–655. doi: 10.1016/s1350-4533(01)00093-5

Martufi, G., Martino, E. S. D., Amon, C. H., Muluk, S. C. and Finol, E. A. (2009). Three-Dimensional Geometrical Characterization of Abdominal Aortic Aneurysms: Image-Based Wall Thickness Distribution. *Journal of Biomechanical Engineering*, *131*(6). doi: 10.1115/1.3127256

Martufi, G., Satriano, A., Moore, R. D., Vorp, D. A. and Martino, E. S. D. (2015). Local Quantification of Wall Thickness and Intraluminal Thrombus Offer Insight into the Mechanical Properties of the Aneurysmal Aorta. *Annals of Biomedical Engineering*, *43*(8), 1759–1771. doi: 10.1007/s10439-014-1222-2

Michel, J.-B., Martin-Ventura, J.-L., Egido, J., Sakalihasan, N., Treska, V., Lindholt, J. and Swedenborg, J. (2010). Novel aspects of the pathogenesis of aneurysms of the abdominal aorta in humans. *Cardiovascular Research*, *90*(1), 18–27. doi: 10.1093/cvr/cvq337

Mix, D. S., Yang, L., Johnson, C. C., Couper, N., Zarras, B., Arabadjis, I., Trakimas L. E., Stoner M. C., Day S. W. and Richards, M. S. (2017). Detecting Regional Stiffness Changes in Aortic Aneurysmal Geometries Using Pressure-Normalized Strain. *Ultrasound in Medicine & Biology*, *43*(10), 2372–2394. doi: 10.1016/j.ultrasmedbio.2017.06.002

Niestrawska, J. A., Viertler, C., Regitnig, P., Cohnert, T. U., Sommer, G. and Holzapfel, G. A. (2016). Microstructure and mechanics of healthy and aneurysmatic abdominal aortas: experimental analysis and modelling. *Journal of the Royal Society Interface*, *13*(124), 20160620. doi: 10.1098/rsif.2016.0620

Nilsson, O., Hultgren, R. and Letterstål, A. (2017). Perceived learning needs of patients with abdominal aortic aneurysm. *Journal of Vascular Nursing*, 35(1), 4–11. doi: 10.1016/j.jvn.2016.08.003

O'Donnell T. F. X., Landon B. E., and Schermerhorn M. L. (2019). AAA Screening Should Be Expanded. *Circulation* 140 (11):889-890. doi: 10.1161/CIRCULATIONAHA.119.041116.

Orgera, G., Tipaldi, M. A., Laurino, F., Lucatelli, P., Rebonato, A., Paraskevopoulos, I., Rossi M. and Krokidis, M. (2019). Techniques and future perspectives for the prevention and treatment of endoleaks after endovascular repair of abdominal aortic aneurysms. *Insights into Imaging*, 10(1). doi: 10.1186/s13244-019-0774-y

Parikh, S. A., Gomez, R., Thirugnanasambandam, M., Chauhan, S. S., Oliveira, V. D., Muluk, S. C., Eskandari M. K. and Finol, E. A. (2018). Decision Tree Based Classification of Abdominal Aortic Aneurysms Using Geometry Quantification Measures. *Annals of Biomedical Engineering*, 46(12), 2135–2147. doi: 10.1007/s10439-018-02116-w

Patel M. I., Hardman D. T., Fisher C. M., and Appleberg M. (1995). Current views on the pathogenesis of abdominal aortic aneurysms. *J Am Coll Surg* 181 (4):371-82.

Piazza, R., Condino, S., Alberti, A., Berchiolli, R. N., Coppi, G., Gesi, M., Ferrari V., and Ferrari, M. (2017). Design of a sensorized guiding catheter for in situ laser fenestration of endovascular stent. *Computer Assisted Surgery*, 22(1), 27–38. doi: 10.1080/24699322.2017.1358403

Polzer, S. and Gasser, T. C. (2015). Biomechanical rupture risk assessment of abdominal aortic aneurysms based on a novel probabilistic rupture risk index. *Journal of the Royal Society Interface*, 12(113), 20150852. doi: 10.1098/rsif.2015.0852

Polzer, S., Gasser, T. C., Vlachovský, R., Kubíček, L., Lambert, L., Man, V., Novák, Slažanský M., K. Burša J. and Staffa, R. (2020). Biomechanical indices are more sensitive than diameter in predicting rupture of asymptomatic abdominal aortic aneurysms. *Journal of Vascular Surgery*, 71(2). doi: 10.1016/j.jvs.2019.03.051

Powell, J. and Sweeting, M. (2014). Endovascular or Open Repair Strategy for Ruptured Abdominal Aortic Aneurysm: Thirty-Day Outcomes from

IMPROVE Randomised Trial. *Journal of Vascular Surgery*, *59*(5), 1470. doi: 10.1016/j.jvs.2014.03.264

Raghavan, M. and Vorp, D. A. (2000). Toward a biomechanical tool to evaluate, rupture potential of abdominal aortic aneurysm: identification of a finite strain constitutive model and evaluation of its applicability. *Journal of Biomechanics*, *33*(4), 475–482. doi: 10.1016/s0021-9290(99)00201-8

Raghavan, M. L., Kratzberg, J., Tolosa, E. M. C. D., Hanaoka, M. M., Walker, P. and Silva, E. S. D. (2006). Regional distribution of wall thickness and failure properties of human abdominal aortic aneurysm. *Journal of Biomechanics*, *39*(16), 3010–3016. doi: 10.1016/j.jbiomech.2005.10.021

Ramadan, A., Al-Omran, M. and Verma, S. (2017). The putative role of autophagy in the pathogenesis of abdominal aortic aneurysms. *Atherosclerosis*, *257*, 288–296. doi: 10.1016/j.atherosclerosis.2017.01.017

Raut, S. S., Chandra, S., Shum, J., Washington, C. B., Muluk, S. C., Finol, E. A. and Rodriguez, J. F. (2013). Biological, Geometric and Biomechanical Factors Influencing Abdominal Aortic Aneurysm Rupture Risk: A Comprehensive Review. *Recent Patents on Medical Imaging*, *3*(1), 44–59. doi: 10.2174/1877613211303010006

Raut, S. S., Liu, P. and Finol, E. A. (2015). An approach for patient-specific multi-domain vascular mesh generation featuring spatially varying wall thickness modeling. *Journal of Biomechanics*, *48*(10), 1972–1981. doi: 10.1016/j.jbiomech.2015.04.006

Reeps, C., Maier, A., Pelisek, J., Härtl, F., Grabher-Meier, V., Wall, W. A. Essler H., Eckstein H. and Gee, M. W. (2012). Measuring and modeling patient-specific distributions of material properties in abdominal aortic aneurysm wall. *Biomechanics and Modeling in Mechanobiology*, *12*(4), 717–733. doi: 10.1007/s10237-012-0436-1

Robert, M., Juillière, Y., Gabet, A., Kownator, S. and Olié, V. (2017). Time trends in hospital admissions and mortality due to abdominal aortic aneurysms in France, 2002–2013. *International Journal of Cardiology*, *234*, 28–32. doi: 10.1016/j.ijcard.2017.02.089

Galarreta, S. R. D., Cazón, A., Antón, R. and Finol, E. A. (2016). A Methodology for Verifying Abdominal Aortic Aneurysm Wall Stress. *Journal of Biomechanical Engineering, 139*(1). doi: 10.1115/1.4034710

Rouet, L., Dufour, C., Billon, A. C. and Bredahl, K. (2019). CT and 3D-ultrasound registration for spatial comparison of post-EVAR abdominal aortic aneurysm measurements: A cross-sectional study. *Computerized Medical Imaging and Graphics, 73*, 49–59. doi: 10.1016/j.compmedimag.2019.02.004

Rudarakanchana, N. and Powell, J. T. (2013). Advances in Imaging and Surveillance of AAA: When, How, How Often? *Progress in Cardiovascular Diseases, 56*(1), 7–12. doi: 10.1016/j.pcad.2013.05.006.

Sano M., T. Sasaki, Hirakawa S., Sakabe J., Ogawa M., Baba S., Zaima N., Tanaka H., Inuzuka K., Yamamoto N., Setou M., Sato K., Konno H. and N. Unno. (2014). Lymphangiogenesis and angiogenesis in abdominal aortic aneurysm. *PLoS One* 9 (3):e89830. doi: 10.1371/journal.pone.0089830.

Schmitz-Rixen, T., Keese, M., Hakimi, M., Peters, A., Böckler, D., Nelson, K. and Grundmann, R. T. (2016). Ruptured abdominal aortic aneurysm—epidemiology, predisposing factors, and biology. *Langenbecks Archives of Surgery, 401*(3), 275–288. doi: 10.1007/s00423-016-1401-8

Shang, E. K., Nathan, D. P., Fairman, R. M., Woo, E. Y., Wang, G. J., Gorman, R. C. and Jackson, B. M. (2013). Local Wall Thickness in Finite Element Models Improves Prediction of Abdominal Aortic Aneurysm Growth. *Journal of Vascular Surgery, 57*(5). doi: 10.1016/j.jvs.2013.02.137

Shum J., Martufi G., Di Martino E., Washington B. C., Grisafi J., Muluk S. C. and Finol A. E. (2011). Quantitative assessment of abdominal aortic aneurysm geometry. *Ann Biomed Eng* 39 (1):277-86. doi: 10.1007/s10439-010-0175-3.

Speelman, L., Bohra, A., Bosboom, E. M. H., Schurink, G. W. H., Vosse, F. N. V. D., Makaroun, M. S. and Vorp, D. A. (2006). Effects of Wall Calcifications in Patient-Specific Wall Stress Analyses of Abdominal

Aortic Aneurysms. *Journal of Biomechanical Engineering, 129*(1), 105–109. doi: 10.1115/1.2401189

Speelman, L., Schurink, G. W. H., Bosboom, E. M. H., Buth, J., Breeuwer, M., Vosse, F. N. V. D. and Jacobs, M. H. (2010). The mechanical role of thrombus on the growth rate of an abdominal aortic aneurysm. *Journal of Vascular Surgery, 51*(1), 19–26. doi: 10.1016/j.jvs.2009.08.075

Sprynger M., Willems M., Van Damme H., Drieghe B., J. C. Wautrecht J. C. and Moonen M. (2019). Screening Program of Abdominal Aortic Aneurysm. *Angiology* 70:407-413.

Stevens, R. R. F., Grytsan, A., Biasetti, J., Roy, J., Liljeqvist, M. Lv Gasser, T. C. (2017). Biomechanical changes during abdominal aortic aneurysm growth. *PlosOne, 12*(11).doi: 10.1371/journal.pone.0187421

Takagi, H., Ando, T. and Umemoto, T. (2017). Abdominal Aortic Aneurysm Screening Reduces All-Cause Mortality: Make Screening Great Again. *Angiology, 69*(3), 205–211. doi: 10.1177/0003319717693107

Tang, A., Kauffmann, C., Tremblay-Paquet, S., Elkouri, S., Steinmetz, O., Morin-Roy, F., Cloutier-Gill L. and Soulez, G. (2014). Morphologic evaluation of ruptured and symptomatic abdominal aortic aneurysm by three-dimensional modeling. *Journal of Vascular Surgery, 59*(4). doi: 10.1016/j.jvs.2013.10.097

Tang, W., Yao, L., Hoogeveen, R. C., Alonso, A., Couper, D. J., Lutsey, P. L., Steenson C. C., Folsom, Guan W., Hunter D. W., Lederle F. A. and Folsom A. R. (2018). The Association of Biomarkers of Inflammation and Extracellular Matrix Degradation with the Risk of Abdominal Aortic Aneurysm: The ARIC Study. *Angiology, 70*(2), 130–140. doi: 10.1177/0003319718785278.

Tarafdar S. A., and Ganno M. X., (2017). Abdominal aortic aneurysm. *InnovAiT Journal* (0):1-7.

Tierney, Á. P., Callanan, A. and Mcgloughlin, T. M. (2012). Use of Regional Mechanical Properties of Abdominal Aortic Aneurysms to Advance Finite Element Modeling of Rupture Risk. *ASME 2012 Summer Bioengineering Conference, Parts A and B.* doi: 10.1115/sbc2012-80181

Urrutia, J., Roy, A., Raut, S. S., Antón, R., Muluk, S. C. and Finol, E. A. (2018). Geometric surrogates of abdominal aortic aneurysm wall mechanics. *Medical Engineering & Physics*, *59*, 43–49. doi: 10.1016/j.medengphy.2018.06.007

Villard, C. and Hultgren, R. (2018). Abdominal aortic aneurysm: Sex differences. *Maturitas*, *109*, 63–69. doi: 10.1016/j.maturitas.2017.12.012

Vorp, D. A., Raghavan, M. L., Muluk, S. C., Makaroun, M. S., Steed, D. L., Shapiro, Rv Webster, M. W. (1996). Wall Strength and Stiffness of Aneurysmal and Nonaneurysmal Abdominal Aorta. *Annals of the New York Academy of Sciences*, *800*(1 The Abdominal), 274–276. doi: 10.1111/j.1749-6632.1996.tb33330.x

Vorp, D. A., Raghavan, M. and Webster, M. W. (1998). Mechanical wall stress in abdominal aortic aneurysm: Influence of diameter and asymmetry. *Journal of Vascular Surgery*, *27*(4), 632–639. doi: 10.1016/s0741-5214(98)70227-7

Vu, K.-N., Kaitoukov, Y., Morin-Roy, F., Kauffmann, C., Giroux, M.-F., Thérasse, É. and Tang, A. (2014). Rupture signs on computed tomography, treatment, and outcome of abdominal aortic aneurysms. *Insights into Imaging*, *5*(3), 281–293. doi: 10.1007/s13244-014-0327-3

Wang, Y., Krishna, S., Walker, P. J., Norman, P. and Golledge, J. (2013). Transforming growth factor-β and abdominal aortic aneurysms. *Cardiovascular Pathology*, *22*(2), 126–132. doi: 10.1016/j.carpath.2012.07.005

Wanhainen, A., Mani, K. and Golledge, J. (2016). Surrogate Markers of Abdominal Aortic Aneurysm Progression. *Arteriosclerosis, Thrombosis, and Vascular Biology*, *36*(2), 236–244. doi: 10.1161/atvbaha.115.306538

Williams, C. R. and Brooke, B. S. (2017). Effectiveness of open versus endovascular abdominal aortic aneurysm repair in population settings: A systematic review of statewide databases. *Surgery*, *162*(4), 707–720. doi: 10.1016/j.surg.2017.01.014

Wilson, K. A., Lee, A. J., Lee, A. J., Hoskins, P. R., Fowkes, F. R., Ruckley, C. and Bradbury, A. W. (2003). The relationship between aortic wall distensibility and rupture of infrarenal abdominal aortic aneurysm. *Journal of Vascular Surgery*, *37*(1), 112–117. doi: 10.1067/mva.2003.40

Wilson, J. S., Baek, S. and Humphrey, J. D. (2012). Importance of initial aortic properties on the evolving regional anisotropy, stiffness and wall thickness of human abdominal aortic aneurysms. *Journal of the Royal Society Interface*, *9*(74), 2047–2058. doi: 10.1098/rsif.2012.0097

Wilson, J. S., Bersi, M. R., Li, G. and Humphrey, J. D. (2017). Correlation of Wall Microstructure and Heterogeneous Distributions of Strain in Evolving Murine Abdominal Aortic Aneurysms. *Cardiovascular Engineering and Technology*, *8*(2), 193–204. doi: 10.1007/s13239-017-0301-6

Wittek, A., Derwich, W., Fritzen, C. P., Schmitz-Rixen, T. and Blase, C. (2018). Towards non-invasive in vivo characterization of the pathophysiological state and mechanical wall strength of the individual human AAA wall based on 4D ultrasound measurements. *ZAMM - Journal of Applied Mathematics and Mechanics / Zeitschrift Für Angewandte Mathematik Und Mechanik*, *98*(12), 2275–2294. doi: 10.1002/zamm.201700353

Wu, W., Rengarajan, B., Thirugnanasambandam, M., Parikh, S., Gomez, R., Oliveira, V. D., Muluk S. C. and Finol, E. A. (2019). Wall Stress and Geometry Measures in Electively Repaired Abdominal Aortic Aneurysms. *Annals of Biomedical Engineering*, *47*(7), 1611–1625. doi: 10.1007/s10439-019-02261-w

Zeinali-Davarani, S., Raguin, L. G., Vorp, D. A. and Baek, S. (2010). Identification of in vivo material and geometric parameters of a human aorta: toward patient-specific modeling of abdominal aortic aneurysm. *Biomechanics and Modeling in Mechanobiology*, *10*(5), 689–699. doi: 10.1007/s10237-010-0266-y

Zhou, R., Yazdi, A. S., Menu, P. and Tschopp, J. (2010). A role for mitochondria in NLRP3 inflammasome activation. *Nature*, *469*(7329), 221–225. doi: 10.1038/nature09663

Editor's Contact Information

Amer Harky
MBChB, MRCS, MSc
StR Cardiothoracic Surgery
Liverpool Heart and Chest Hospital

INDEX

A

abdominal aortic aneurysm, ix, 33, 35, 36, 37, 38, 40, 41, 42, 43, 45, 46, 47, 48, 49, 50, 51, 52, 53, 57, 58, 59, 60, 65, 68, 74, 76, 90, 92, 94, 102, 109, 110, 111, 133, 134, 136, 137, 138, 139, 140, 141, 142, 143, 144, 145, 146, 147
adventitia, 3, 7, 12, 20
aetiology, 2, 3, 8, 24, 33
age, 2, 73, 74, 113, 114, 127, 128
anatomy, viii, 35, 64, 66, 67, 72, 73, 90, 128, 131
aneurysm, v, vii, viii, ix, 1, 2, 3, 4, 5, 7, 8, 9, 10, 11, 14, 16, 17, 20, 22, 23, 27, 28, 29, 30, 33, 34, 35, 36, 37, 38, 39, 40, 41, 42, 43, 44, 45, 46, 47, 49, 50, 51, 52, 53, 54, 55, 57, 58, 59, 60, 63, 64, 65, 66, 67, 68, 70, 71, 72, 73, 74, 76, 77, 80, 81, 82, 83, 85, 86, 87, 88, 89, 90, 91, 93, 94, 96, 97, 99, 100, 101, 102, 103, 104, 105, 110, 111, 112, 113, 115, 116, 119, 121, 125, 130, 131, 132, 133, 134, 135, 136, 137, 138, 139, 140, 141, 142, 143, 144, 145, 146, 147
angiogenesis, 8, 29, 57, 115, 144
angiography, 75, 129, 139
angiotensin II, 7, 23, 36, 39, 46, 55
antigen, 4, 6, 11, 13, 15, 18, 19, 23, 25, 46
aorta, vii, ix, 1, 2, 3, 6, 10, 16, 30, 32, 35, 57, 66, 68, 71, 74, 75, 78, 79, 89, 91, 109, 110, 111, 113, 115, 116, 117, 121, 131, 141, 147
aortic aneurysm, vii, viii, 2, 3, 6, 8, 9, 10, 11, 12, 14, 15, 18, 19, 21, 24, 28, 29, 30, 31, 33, 34, 35, 36, 38, 39, 42, 43, 44, 47, 53, 55, 56, 57, 58, 60, 63, 64, 65, 66, 67, 68, 70, 71, 72, 73, 74, 76, 77, 80, 82, 83, 88, 90, 91, 92, 93, 94, 95, 96, 97, 100, 101, 137, 140
apoptosis, viii, 2, 4, 9, 11, 17, 30
arteries, 68, 70, 82, 89, 115, 131
artery, ix, 48, 64, 70, 74, 75, 76, 80, 84, 90, 91, 101, 131, 132
arthritis, 23, 26, 41
assessment, 98, 104, 118, 129, 144
asymmetry, 113, 114, 126, 146
asymptomatic, viii, 1, 2, 76, 110, 114, 119, 142
atherosclerosis, 3, 4, 7, 8, 12, 14, 19, 20, 26, 31, 35, 39, 43, 44, 48, 50, 143

atherosclerotic plaque, 13, 17, 27, 44, 45, 50, 59
autoimmune disease, 22, 23, 24
autoimmune diseases, 22, 23, 24

B

basophils, 11, 15, 19, 42
biomechanical parameters, ix, 110, 114, 121, 134
blood, viii, 3, 5, 6, 7, 11, 14, 25, 27, 30, 38, 52, 54, 64, 66, 69, 70, 71, 75, 113, 116, 117, 121, 123, 124, 125, 131
blood flow, viii, 3, 14, 30, 64, 66, 69, 70, 71, 75, 116, 124, 125
blood pressure, 38, 113, 117, 121, 123, 131
bone, 11, 18, 22, 39, 101
bone marrow, 11, 18, 22, 39

C

calcification, 3, 115, 117, 120, 132, 136
cancer, 26, 29, 37, 57
cardiovascular disease(s), 2, 12, 28, 43, 45, 57, 65, 98, 128
catheter, viii, 63, 142
CD8+, 15, 17, 45
challenges, 91, 102, 135
chemokine receptor, 7, 17, 39
chemokines, 6, 7, 19, 29, 33
clinical trials, ix, 64, 65, 87
collagen, 3, 4, 6, 7, 9, 29, 32, 37, 111, 113, 115, 120, 121, 123, 124
complement, viii, 2, 31, 59, 60
compliance, 92, 111, 113
complications, 67, 69, 77, 80, 81, 90, 135
computational fluid dynamics, 73, 75, 82, 87, 89, 98, 101
computed tomography, 119, 129, 135, 136, 140, 146
connective tissue, 4, 12, 66, 115

control group, 16, 19, 24
correlation(s), 12, 26, 30, 48, 113, 119, 123, 128
cost, 83, 112, 129
CT scan, 82, 119, 138
cytokines, 3, 4, 5, 6, 8, 11, 12, 13, 15, 16, 17, 19, 20, 22, 25, 26, 27, 28, 30, 32, 33, 115

D

deaths, 2, 65, 71
deficiency, 10, 14, 16, 18, 27, 54, 55
deformation, 116, 122, 125
degeneration, viii, 2, 4, 12, 26, 28, 115, 124
degradation, 5, 8, 9, 10, 12, 13, 18, 22, 23, 27, 28, 30, 42, 111, 113, 115, 120, 123, 124
dendritic cell, 4, 7, 25, 44, 115
deposition, 4, 6, 8, 31, 116, 136
diabetes, 24, 26, 52, 53, 79, 128
dilation, 2, 19, 28, 48, 115
diseases, 16, 20, 28, 35, 37, 50, 78, 92
distribution, 75, 111, 116, 120, 122, 124, 125, 139, 143
diversity, 22, 49, 54
drugs, 8, 22, 106

E

ECM, 5, 6, 8, 9, 11, 22, 29, 30, 32, 115, 116
ECM degradation, 5, 7, 30, 115
elastin, 4, 7, 9, 18, 22, 29, 38, 42, 111, 113, 115, 120, 124
emergency, viii, ix, 1, 64, 69, 72, 80, 131
engineering, ix, 64, 102, 111
environment(s), 5, 6, 82, 83, 124
eosinophils, 11, 12, 15, 19, 42
evidence, 5, 8, 13, 16, 17, 18, 27, 29, 30, 31, 72, 82
evolution, 68, 77, 87

exposure, 19, 20, 22, 129, 130
extracellular matrix, 5, 57, 115, 123, 124

F

family history, 126, 127, 128
fibers, 113, 121, 123
fibroblasts, 3, 29, 42
fluid, ix, 3, 64, 78, 83, 98, 101, 102, 107
formation, vii, 4, 7, 9, 10, 11, 12, 14, 17, 19, 20, 22, 23, 24, 27, 29, 30, 32, 35, 36, 39, 40, 42, 45, 46, 51, 55, 58, 82, 83, 113, 116, 123, 126

G

genes, 17, 51, 60
geometrical indices, ix, 110, 118, 119, 120
geometry, 87, 112, 114, 118, 119, 126, 129, 135, 144
giant cell arteritis, 13, 14, 44
growth, ix, 12, 19, 28, 30, 32, 37, 65, 71, 82, 110, 115, 116, 118, 120, 123, 124, 127, 130, 132, 138, 139, 145, 146
growth factor, 32, 37, 146
growth rate, 118, 123, 124, 145
guidelines, 88, 110, 137

H

health, ix, 5, 64, 110, 113, 114, 126, 127, 128, 134, 135
history, ix, 72, 110, 113, 114, 127
HLA, 23, 24, 25, 51, 52
host, 11, 15, 25, 40, 50
human, 6, 11, 12, 14, 17, 20, 21, 23, 31, 32, 37, 40, 42, 43, 45, 46, 49, 50, 59, 96, 115, 116, 143, 147
hybrid, 67, 96, 97, 99
hypertension, 6, 57, 79

I

IFN, 5, 6, 12, 15, 16, 17, 20, 27, 30, 44, 45
IL-13, 11, 12, 15, 16, 20, 21, 44
IL-17, 15, 16, 20, 45
image, 83, 104, 117, 129, 130, 131, 135
images, 119, 123, 135
imaging, 48, 109, 110, 111, 119, 124, 128, 129, 130, 132, 134, 135, 137, 138, 139, 140, 141, 142, 143, 144, 146
immune response, 4, 6, 9, 13, 21, 22, 26, 43, 54
immune system, 3, 4, 13, 16, 25, 115
immunity, 3, 6, 11, 13, 21, 26, 35, 39, 50
immunoglobulin, viii, 2, 19, 25, 44, 59
immunoglobulins, 4, 19, 20, 36
immunopathology, v, vii, viii, 1, 2, 3, 4, 11
immunotherapy, viii, 2, 27
in vitro, 37, 59, 86, 98
incidence, viii, 10, 26, 43, 64
induction, 17, 58, 116
infection, 50, 72, 135
inflammasome, 22, 23, 51, 147
inflammation, 2, 4, 5, 6, 7, 14, 25, 30, 31, 34, 35, 37, 38, 39, 40, 41, 43, 45, 49, 52, 115, 124, 139, 145
inflammatory cells, viii, 2, 3, 9
inflammatory disease, 20, 34, 51
inflammatory responses, 6, 8, 17, 40, 45
inhibition, 7, 17, 31, 39
injury, 7, 8, 59
integrity, viii, 2, 3, 33
interferon, 5, 44, 45
intervention, ix, 2, 54, 64, 74, 75, 78, 79, 87, 97, 132, 134
intima, 3, 14, 43
Ireland, 36, 55, 105, 106
ischemia, 67, 81, 86, 88, 89, 91, 103

J

Jordan, 53, 95, 106, 107

L

lead, viii, ix, 2, 8, 9, 13, 22, 25, 27, 28, 33, 64, 69, 70, 78, 92, 113, 123, 131
lesions, 12, 14, 17, 19, 75
life-style and health factors, 110
ligand, 22, 23, 25
lumen, 3, 73, 75, 79, 117, 125
lymphocytes, 9, 20, 30, 36, 115
lymphoid, 18, 19, 20, 47, 49, 50

M

macrophages, 4, 5, 6, 7, 8, 9, 10, 12, 13, 14, 16, 17, 19, 25, 27, 30, 33, 36, 37, 48, 58, 115
majority, 10, 18, 21
management, vii, viii, 8, 54, 63, 71, 73, 87, 90, 95, 96, 106, 107, 111, 112, 114, 130, 132, 137
Marfan syndrome, 28, 29, 55, 56
mast cells, 3, 4, 11, 15, 19, 42, 48
matrix, 4, 5, 9, 12, 28, 29, 31, 36, 41, 57, 58, 59, 111, 115, 116
matrix metalloproteinase, 4, 5, 29, 36, 41, 57, 58, 59
measurement, 122, 129, 138
measurements, 129, 138, 144, 147
media, 3, 4, 12, 115
medical, ix, 54, 64, 70, 98, 100, 102, 130, 133
mellitus, 24, 26, 53
memory, 15, 17, 19
meta-analysis, 53, 73, 89, 90, 106
metalloproteinase, 41, 57, 111, 115

MFM, ix, 64, 70, 71, 72, 73, 74, 75, 76, 77, 78, 79, 80, 81, 82, 83, 86, 107
MHC, 6, 13, 23
mice, 7, 10, 12, 16, 17, 19, 21, 22, 28, 32, 35, 36, 38, 39, 43, 45, 46, 50, 54
migration, 3, 7, 135
MMP, 8, 9, 10, 11, 14, 16, 17, 26, 27, 29, 31, 33, 36
MMP-2, 8, 9, 10, 14, 16, 27, 29, 31
MMP-3, 30, 33
MMP-9, 8, 9, 10, 12, 16, 26, 27, 29, 31
MMPs, 5, 22, 28, 29, 31, 116
modelling, 28, 60, 100, 141
models, 6, 7, 10, 11, 12, 14, 15, 16, 20, 21, 26, 29, 31, 33, 71, 75, 83, 119, 121, 122, 123, 126, 136
molecules, viii, 1, 2, 8, 23, 30, 32, 33, 35
morbidity, vii, 1, 65, 66, 72, 76, 79
morphology, v, ix, 43, 109, 110, 114, 115, 129
mortality, vii, viii, 1, 2, 7, 16, 18, 26, 64, 65, 66, 67, 69, 72, 76, 77, 79, 93, 110, 118, 127, 128, 131, 134, 135, 143
mortality rate, 2, 67, 69, 110, 127, 134, 135
MRI, 129, 130, 135
multilayer stent, 64, 73, 80, 88, 89, 90, 91, 92, 94

N

neutrophils, 4, 9, 10, 11, 16, 30, 40
nitric oxide, 4, 6, 30, 59
nitric oxide synthase, 6, 30, 59

O

oxidative stress, 7, 10, 38
oxygen, 30, 59, 124

Index

P

parallel, viii, 33, 64, 69
pathogenesis, 3, 5, 20, 35, 36, 38, 41, 42, 43, 48, 51, 52, 58, 141, 142, 143
pathogens, 6, 13, 15
pathology, vii, 13, 73, 90
pathophysiology, vii, 2, 3, 11, 16, 18, 22, 24, 26, 33, 136
pathway, 14, 21, 22, 23, 25, 26, 32, 43, 52, 54, 55, 60
pathways, 28, 30, 32, 80
peptides, 7, 28, 38, 42
perfusion, viii, 64, 68, 71, 75, 79, 86, 91, 94
phagocytosis, 6, 8, 9
phenotype, 5, 17, 20, 46
phenotypes, 5, 6, 7, 14, 21, 36
physiology, 6, 111, 134
plaque, 4, 20, 30, 45
polarization, 37, 38, 46
polymorphisms, 22, 24, 60
population, 2, 15, 19, 21, 24, 52, 53, 146
positive correlation, 118, 119, 123, 124, 128
positive feedback, 7, 10, 30
preservation, 10, 80, 82, 83
prevention, 8, 26, 91, 116, 142
probability, 117, 118, 120, 132
pro-inflammatory, 3, 5, 6, 26, 115
proliferation, 7, 12, 14, 17, 21, 25
protection, 10, 21, 28, 45
proteins, 11, 25, 28, 29, 32, 51, 116

R

Ramadan, 110, 114, 143
reactive oxygen, 4, 40, 58
receptor, 5, 6, 7, 22, 23, 25, 33, 35, 37, 39, 42, 50, 51
receptors, 3, 4, 11, 19, 20, 21, 28, 33, 50
recognition, 18, 22, 23, 33, 50
reconstruction, 121, 129, 137
recovery, viii, 63, 66
remodelling, 3, 5, 6, 8, 9, 12, 30
repair, vii, viii, ix, 1, 6, 8, 35, 38, 63, 64, 65, 66, 67, 68, 69, 72, 73, 74, 76, 78, 81, 82, 86, 87, 88, 89, 90, 91, 92, 93, 94, 95, 96, 97, 100, 106, 107, 110, 112, 118, 124, 127, 128, 130, 131, 133, 134, 135, 140, 141, 142, 146
response, viii, 2, 4, 9, 15, 16, 17, 25, 26, 27, 29, 42, 46, 52, 55, 58, 111, 121, 122, 125
rheumatoid arthritis, 24, 26, 28, 51, 53, 54, 55
risk, viii, ix, 2, 25, 28, 30, 32, 50, 63, 64, 66, 67, 68, 70, 72, 74, 79, 86, 94, 110, 112, 114, 115, 116, 117, 118, 119, 120, 121, 123, 124, 127, 129, 130, 133, 134, 135, 137, 138, 141, 142
root, vii, 1, 3
Royal Society, 141, 142, 147

S

safety, 73, 82, 86, 87
secrete, 11, 17, 18
secretion, viii, 1, 6, 9, 12, 16, 20, 115
serine, 9, 11, 41
serum, 10, 16, 19
shape, 114, 116, 118, 119
shear, ix, 64, 70, 71, 75, 83, 85, 122
showing, 21, 84, 111, 120, 125
signalling, 6, 7, 8, 21, 22, 23, 28, 30
signals, 11, 27, 116
Singapore, 63, 97, 98, 100, 101, 102, 103
smoking, 113, 114, 127, 128, 135
smooth muscle, viii, 2, 3, 37, 45, 47, 113, 115, 116, 124, 136
smooth muscle cells, viii, 2, 3, 37, 45, 113, 115, 116, 124
solution, 26, 65, 72, 126
species, 4, 11, 40, 58, 59
spinal cord, 35, 81, 89, 91

stability, 9, 59, 117
state(s), viii, 1, 7, 26, 75, 89, 147
stent, viii, 63, 64, 68, 69, 70, 73, 74, 77, 78, 79, 80, 82, 83, 86, 87, 88, 90, 91, 92, 93, 94, 95, 100, 131, 135, 142
stress, ix, 10, 33, 64, 65, 70, 71, 75, 83, 85, 111, 112, 113, 114, 116, 117, 118, 120, 121, 122, 123, 124, 125, 126, 136, 137, 138, 139, 146
stroke, 67, 71, 92
structure, 3, 32, 101, 117, 125, 129, 132, 141
style, 110, 113, 126
Sun, 12, 43, 57, 58, 97
suppression, 10, 19, 27
surgical intervention, vii, 67, 72, 106
survival, 26, 71, 73
susceptibility, 17, 23, 51
syndrome, 19, 28, 48, 52
systemic lupus erythematosus, 23, 26, 52, 53, 55

T

T cell(s), 4, 12, 13, 14, 15, 16, 17, 18, 19, 20, 21, 23, 25, 26, 45, 46, 48, 53
T lymphocytes, 4, 12, 33, 45, 54
TAA, viii, ix, 4, 8, 12, 18, 20, 22, 28, 32, 63, 64, 66, 67, 68, 77, 83
target, 7, 17, 21, 26, 30, 31, 81
techniques, viii, ix, 35, 64, 69, 88, 94, 111, 134
technology, ix, 64, 70, 82, 87, 102
testing, 32, 72, 83, 98
TEVAR, viii, ix, 63, 64, 66, 67, 69, 86, 89
TGF, 6, 8, 15, 18, 27, 28, 29, 33, 47, 55, 56, 57, 115, 116
therapeutic targets, 7, 10, 27

therapeutics, 2, 8, 23, 30, 51, 55, 98
therapy, 19, 36, 51, 55, 80, 87
thrombus, 9, 10, 42, 71, 82, 83, 101, 113, 114, 115, 116, 120, 121, 124, 132, 136, 145
tissue, 4, 5, 6, 7, 8, 9, 10, 16, 31, 32, 57, 58, 59, 111, 113, 117, 121, 122, 123, 125, 130, 135, 136
TLR, 6, 21, 23
TNF, 6, 8, 11, 15, 22, 27, 30, 54, 55
TNF-α, 6, 8, 11, 15, 22, 27, 30, 54
transcription, 22, 30, 38
transforming growth factor, 6, 55, 56, 60, 115, 116
treatment, ix, 26, 33, 57, 64, 65, 66, 67, 69, 70, 71, 72, 73, 74, 75, 76, 77, 78, 79, 82, 85, 86, 87, 88, 89, 90, 91, 92, 93, 94, 96, 97, 99, 100, 103, 104, 105, 110, 111, 116, 126, 128, 130, 131, 133, 134, 142, 146
treatment methods, 86, 111, 126, 128, 131, 133
trial, 81, 82, 86, 87, 134, 135
triggers, 22, 41, 42
tumor, 53, 54, 57, 99, 103

U

ultrasound, 103, 128, 137, 140, 144, 147
uniform, 33, 112, 113, 123, 126, 127
United States (USA), 48, 65, 128, 139

V

vascular diseases, vii, 1, 4
vasculature, 9, 26, 28, 30
velocity, 71, 84, 85, 87
vessels, 69, 70, 71, 75, 84, 93, 115